MW01703065

THE ADDICT'S GUIDE TO RECOVERY

THE ADDICT'S GUIDE TO RECOVERY

The Addict's Guide to the Universe: Book One

FREEDOM
RECOVERY
PRESS

The Addict's Guide to Recovery

www.theaddictsguidetotheuniverse.com

Publisher's Cataloging-in-Publication data

Names: Sussman, Emily, author. | Larson, J. E., illustrator.
Title: The addict's guide to recovery : the addict's guide to the universe , book one / Emily Sussman; illustrated by J.E. Larson.
Series: The Addict's Guide to the Universe
Description: Granger, IN: Freedom Recovery Press, 2023.
Identifiers: LCCN: 2023910532 | ISBN: 979-8-9884786-0-7 (paperback) | 979-8-9884786-1-4 (epub)
Subjects: LCSH Substance abuse--Treatment. | Compulsive behavior--Treatment. | Recovering alcoholics. | Recovering addicts. | Addicts--Rehabilitation. | Addicts--Psychology. | BISAC SELF-HELP / Substance Abuse & Addictions / General | PSYCHOLOGY / Psychopathology / Addiction
Classification: LCC RC564.29 .S87 2023 | DDC 616.86/0651--dc23

Ordering Information:
If you are interested in quantity sales for your organization, please contact Emily Sussman at emily@freedomrecoverysb.com.

Illustrations © J. E. Larson
Book design by Bobbi Benson, Wild Ginger Press

For my parents,
Len and Mary Ellen

CONTENTS

ABOUT THE SERIES

As an addiction therapist first and a writer second, my idea to create a series on recovery was borne of frustration. I was trying to provide informational handouts for my clients on the topics we were discussing in group therapy, but I wasn't satisfied with the articles I was digging up on the Internet. Eventually, I started writing my own explanations of the tools and concepts that go along with living in recovery. It occurred to me that if I compiled them into a book, it could help addicts far beyond the confines of my own practice.

Excitement took over, and — addict that I am — I spent the next week feverishly creating a 60-chapter outline, impulsively titling it, "The Addict's Guide to the Universe." A take on Douglas Adams' sci-fi classic, *The Hitchhiker's Guide to the Galaxy*, I wanted the name to convey that there was a fun, cosmic, and truthful way to understand the existential personal journey that goes hand-in-hand with the process of recovery.

That original outline proved too ambitious for one book. Not wanting to overwhelm anyone (especially myself), I've broken it down into several bite-sized chunks. Each volume in the series is written expressly for addicts who want to heal, grow, and understand themselves better, so they can live their best and fullest lives. And while the act of reading a book could never be a substitute for fostering the self-love and loving relationships at the heart of recovery, my hope is that the series provides guidance, insight, and hope to the addicts it attracts.

This first book in the series is an overview of how recovery breaks the cycle of addiction by addressing an addict's deeper, unmet needs for love. The second book will be a practical guide to applying the most important principles of love — what I like to refer to as "recovery superpowers" — to promote peace, freedom, and happiness in day-to-day life. The remainder of the books in the series will cover feelings, relationships, and the process of discovering one's "True Self."

In the bigger picture, I want to offer recovering people an accessible and engaging alternative to all the dry and deadly serious resources in the addiction self-help genre. I know it's possible to articulate the tools and concepts of recovery in a way that's just as hopeful and human as it is honest. Most importantly, I want to make the voice of this series personal and familiar — so that every addict reading it knows they are never alone.

As a byproduct of writing The Addict's Guide to the Universe series, I began producing a podcast of the same name. The best thing about the medium of podcasting is that it's literally given that voice of understanding to addicts, no matter where they happen to be in the world. I have immense gratitude for the listeners who sent me emails of appreciation, which encouraged me to keep going with the project.

Regardless of whether it's received in written or spoken form, I hope that the voice of the series will continue to be a source of comfort and strength for anyone who wants a way out of the isolation and insanity of addiction.

On a personal note, the three years it took to get this first book to publication has been a mirror of my own recovery journey. In order to provide a voice for other addicts, I've had to discover my own, and push myself to make it a strong, clear, and honest one. The project has also forced me to challenge any lingering limiting beliefs I had about myself, and to persevere in a way I never had before. If I hadn't held fast to my faith in the power of love to see me through — that is, the faith I've built over the course of my own recovery — I would have given up many times along the way.

But if I'd had only my own experience in recovery as the basis for writing this series, it would have been an impossible project to undertake. I'm fortunate to have built a career in which I get to spend every day working with and learning from the stories of other recovering addicts. My knowledge of the subject has also been enriched by all the honesty that's been so freely shared with me by my friends and fellows in my own recovery community.

Witnessing the miracle of transformation and rebirth in so many of the addicts I've known, both personally and professionally, has given me the gift of truth. Namely, that even the most hopeless and cynical of addicts can learn to believe in, connect to, and harness the healing power of love in their recovery.

My dear Addict friends, please take heart that no one walks a perfectly straight line on this journey, not even an addiction therapist. But the best thing about staying on the road of recovery is that each honest step you take — no matter how awkward or terrifying — will help you build faith and love within yourself. That faith and love is the best antidote I know of to the fear and shame that feed the mercenary beast that is Your Addict.

And as long as you continue taking steps on this road, I have faith that your life will keep getting better — no matter what.

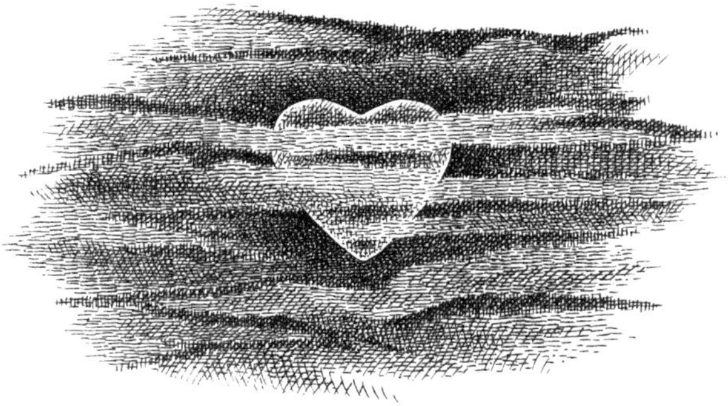

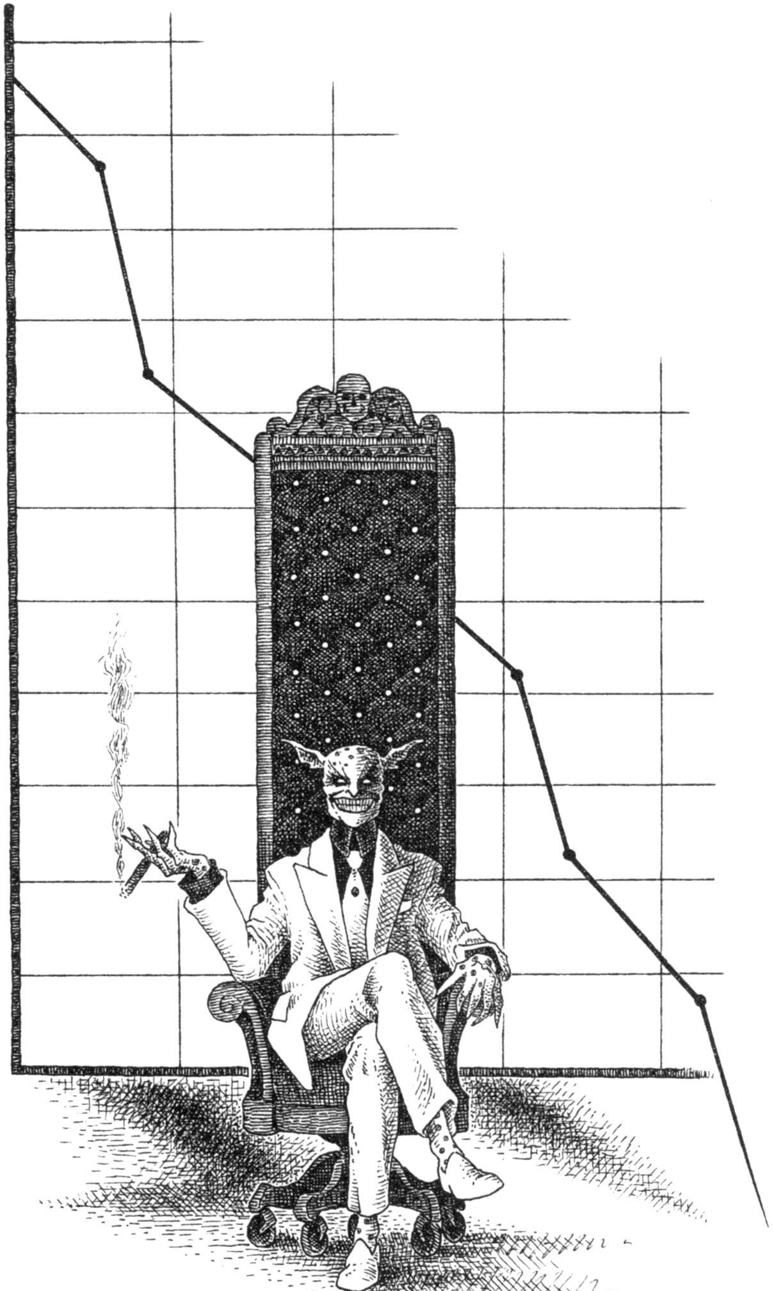

SECTION 1

YOUR ADDICT VS. YOUR TRUE SELF

CHAPTER 1

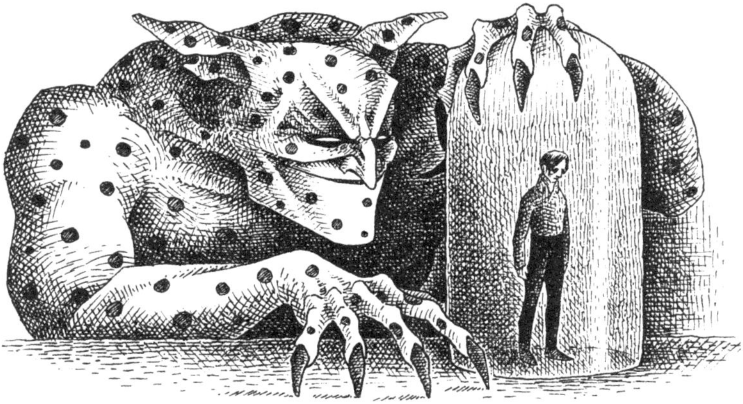

A Few Words About the A-Word

My dear Addict friends, my use of the term "addict" isn't meant to shame you. It's a word I'm using to characterize an entrenched pattern of self-destructive behaviors, along with the thoughts and feelings that prompt them. You can think of Your Addict as a crooked, unhinged, power-hungry personality who's usurped Your True Self as the acting CEO of your life — and it's well on its way to running it into the ground.

Let me assure you that Your Addict isn't who you are, though it definitely exists within you. It's essential to understand that Your Addict has a personality unto itself, which has come to progressively overpower both the free will and the heart and soul of Your True Self.

With that said, my dear Addict friends, I love you. I am you. And I want to help you overthrow Your Addict and put Your True Self back in charge.

Speaking as both an addiction therapist and a recovering addict myself, though, I understand if you're reluctant to wear the scarlet letter "A." Accepting the existence of Your Addict can be a terrifying prospect. Let alone admitting that it's taken complete control of your will, your common sense, and everything you hold dear.

Scary, yes — especially if Your Addict has a long history of keeping you in a stranglehold of secrecy and shame. That's why my objective here will be to help you break through that fear and shame.

As you immerse yourself in the loving little world of this book, please remember that it's just us crazy addicts around here, so there's no need to wear a bag over your head, or even an N95 that conveniently disguises your emotional reactions. By all means, kick off your pinching,

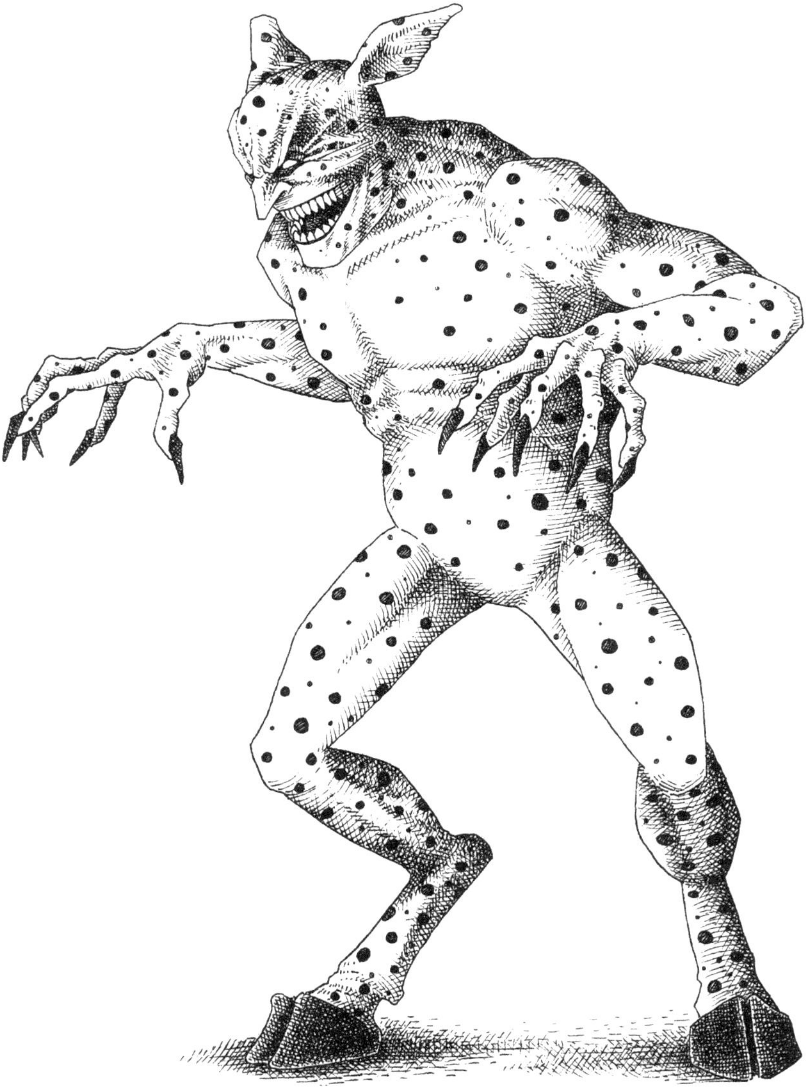

ill-fitting shoes that try so hard to convey, *I'm doing fine and I'm totally normal, really I am!*

Feel free to fling your stinky, callused Addict feet over the warm and fuzzy ottoman of my unconditional acceptance.

My job here is to hold up a mirror to you. One of those incredibly well-lit mirrors, that is, that's going to cut through your cloak of shame and denial, and illuminate your beautiful spirit that lies beneath.

But my agenda of shame-busting isn't just for vanity's sake. It's to help you let go of your fear of seeing the truth about yourself — dark, scary parts and all. That's essential, because the only way you can begin to solve a problem is to acknowledge that there is a problem.

And when it comes to addiction, the problem lies within.

Maybe some of you have already acknowledged the problem that is Your Addict, having long ago surrendered the illusion that you could control your drinking, drugging, or some other addictive behavior. Perhaps you've even gone one further by starting to live in the solution, one terrifying, tenuous, or tedious sober day at a time.

If that's the case, congratulations! Thank you for allowing me to be your guide here on the road of recovery, with nonstop service to peace, freedom, and happiness. Turbulence may be an inevitable part of the journey, but life in recovery is ultimately anything but terrifying, tenuous, or tedious.

But this book is also for all you questioning, might-be addicts out there. Maybe you're seeking insight into that dark and scary part of yourself. Perhaps you have a hunch that you might be a teensy-weensy bit addicted. You've been Dr. Googling search terms like, *does getting three DUIs make me an alcoholic?* or, *can you get addicted to weed?*

If that describes you, chances are, you've already Internet-stumbled upon the eleven criteria for addictive disorders in the principal authority for psychological disorders, the *Diagnostic and Statistical Manual, Fifth Edition* (DSM-V). You've reviewed the criteria dozens of times, hoping to diagnose (or absolve) yourself.

I've paraphrased the DSM-V criteria here:

1. You've been using your drug more often, and for longer amounts of time, than you used to.
2. You're constantly trying to quit or control your use of your drug, without success.
3. You're spending a lot of time thinking about your drug, or recovering from using it.
4. You experience strong cravings for your drug.
5. Your drug prevents you from carrying out your regular responsibilities.
6. Your drug causes problems in your relationships.
7. Your drug prevents you from enjoying the activities you used to enjoy.

8. Your drug puts you in dangerous situations.
9. Your drug is damaging your physical and/or mental health.
10. You have an increased tolerance for your drug, meaning that you have to use more of it, or at a greater intensity or frequency, to get the desired effect.
11. You experience withdrawal symptoms when you aren't using your drug.

These criteria are going to sound eerily familiar to those of you who are ready to get real about what's going on.

I see you, my dear Addict friend, lying prostrate on your bed with a half-empty Dr. Pepper to your left, and a fifth of gin to your right. Your curtains are drawn; it's three in the afternoon. Notifications are piling up on your phone. You've officially withdrawn from life. You're cradling this book with your free hand, the one that's not clutching a bottle. Your pillow is damp with drool, or tears. Maybe both.

You nodded like a bobblehead at all, or nearly all, of the DSM-V criteria. You have no shame admitting this, because you're at a point where shame is beside the point. Even death seems preferable to remaining in Your Addict's clutches another minute.

Or maybe you pored over the DSM-V criteria, considered them, then lobbed your responses back defensively.

Nope, nope, nope, that doesn't describe me! you said, your voice betrayed by a tremor of uncertainty. You couldn't help feeling a chill from the shadow of doubt that's lurking around your ironclad fence of denial.

Obviously, I can't diagnose you from where I'm sitting. But I can tell you that if you're in any amount of emotional pain, or if you've experienced more than a few unpleasant life consequences as a result of Your Addict's insane, out-of-control behavior, then you might want to keep reading. Just in case.

CHAPTER 2

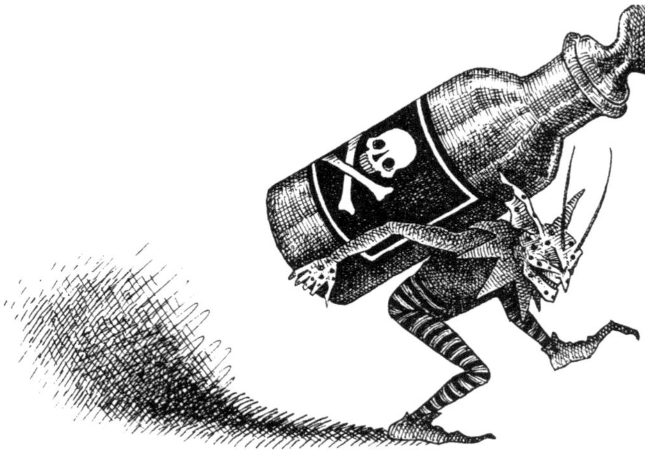

In My Book, a Drug Is a Drug Is a Drug

In my work as an addiction and recovery therapist, I don't just see clients who are addicted to drugs and alcohol. I also work with people who are struggling with compulsive sexual behavior, whether that involves pornography, masturbation, infidelity, visiting sex workers, exhibitionism, or voyeurism. I also treat clients with a history of compulsive gambling, whether that means playing cards at casinos, or online games, or sports betting, or scratch tickets, or any activity in which they're putting money on an outcome.

Alcohol. Gambling. Porn. Pills. Even video games. Whatever it is, it can be to you what I'm calling in this book *a drug*. If you've been using it or doing it compulsively, if it causes problems in your life, and if you're still unable to stop or control it when you realize it's causing problems, then I call it an addiction — to a drug —regardless of what that drug is.

My dear Addict friends, the purpose of this book isn't to analyze the concept of addiction to death. It's to help you understand what it means to live in recovery from it. Because a peaceful, free, and happy life is your birthright, no matter what kind of drug has been enslaving you.

It's baffling to me that this broad, inclusive view on the concept of addictive drugs is a controversial perspective in the world of clinical and research psychology. I know at least one therapist in my area, for instance, who stopped speaking to me after I told him that I treat sexually compulsive behaviors as an addiction. I guess that's because "sexual addiction" still isn't classified in the DSM-V as a psychological disorder.

Let me tell you, though, it's proved incredibly helpful

for my sex addiction clients to be able to put a name to their painful, out-of-control behavior, and to learn how to apply a recovery framework to their lives, the same way other recovering addicts do. Ditto for the video game addicts I've worked with.

As a therapist, I believe in keeping addiction treatment simple. The primary characteristic of addiction is *the problematic loss of control* over one's use of a certain substance, or engagement in a certain behavior. That's why I believe that a drug is a drug is a drug for someone whose brain has been fundamentally changed over weeks, months, or years by the compulsive use or engagement with that drug — as evidenced by their problematic loss of control over it.

So throughout this book, and the others to come in The Addict's Guide to the Universe series, I'm going to call it like it is: *your drug*, based on how it functions in the brain of an addict. Knowing that, maybe now is a good time to recognize which drug *your drug* refers to. Is it alcohol? Pornography? Cocaine? Gambling? Or, perhaps, a combo pack of several different behaviors and/or substances?

The bottom line is that it's not what it is, it's what it does to you that makes it a drug.

Let's keep it simple, shall we? If desire or desperation is telling you (or screaming at you) that you want and need to be free from your drug, then by all means, call yourself an addict. Don't do that to shame yourself, or to take it on as your entire identity. Do it because identifying as an addict who's got to deal with the problem of your drug puts you on the road of the solution: *recovery*.

Do it, my dear Addict friends, because the truth will set you free. You'll see.

Just a note in the name of full disclosure, though: I have not worked with clients in the area of eating disorders, or self-harm, or obsessive-compulsive, ritualistic behaviors, except where those have presented alongside one or more of the substance or behavioral addictions I outlined above. It's not that eating disorders, or self-harm, or OCD don't share many of the same characteristics of addiction. It's simply that those conditions have not been the focus of my professional practice, and you should know that.

CHAPTER 3

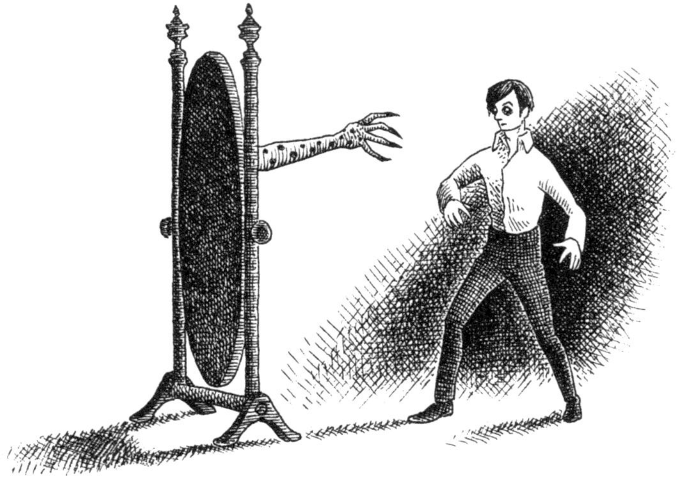

Your Addict Isn't Who You Are

Maybe Your Addict has scaly skin and beady eyes. Maybe it talks all slick and smooth, like a timeshare salesman. Maybe it has a menacing mechanical hand, like Dr. Claw from *Inspector Gadget*.

Personally, I think of My Addict as a toxic ex-boyfriend I've got to stay the hell away from. When life gets dull or difficult, it's tempting to think back wistfully on the good times we shared: the excitement, the pleasure, and the escape from reality. But whenever the thought of my toxic ex starts to seem all sexy and romantic again, I have to remind myself of all the pain he caused me. How he was never okay with me just being myself. How he always wanted me to be someone with no feelings, no needs, and no control over the direction of our relationship. How we went around and around in cycles of codependent craziness, coming up against the same dead ends every time.

I have to remember that even though My Addict may always be lurking around, trying to tempt me to come back, that doesn't mean I should go back. My Addict will always be the same sleazy, loveless asshole he always was, a pretty parasite happy to exploit me for his own selfish gain.

I know that's pretty damning as far as metaphors go, but that's the point. You already know that Your Addict isn't pretty. My point is that Your Addict isn't you.

I've already said that Your Addict has a personality unto itself. The thing about personalities is that they're hard-wired to repeat themselves to produce a desired result: survival. And just like any other personality, Your Addict functions as a pattern of thoughts, feelings, and behaviors that play out in predictable ways, with the goal of keeping itself alive.

Here's where Your Addict's personality goes off the rails, though. It isn't geared toward your survival or well-being. Your Addict's lone objective is to get itself fed with your drug — whether that's alcohol, pills, gambling, pornography, or a good ol' smorgasbord of addictive substances and behaviors.

Feed me! Your Addict hisses at you. *To hell with your well-being and survival!*

Indeed, Your Addict is a hungry beast, and a cunning one at that. It'll pelt you with the perfect storm of self-defeating beliefs, emotional triggers, and situational prompts to use your drug, thereby ensuring not only its survival, but its growth.

Case in point: the characteristic way Your Addict handles problems. (Spoiler: it's terrible with problems.) Your Addict will think and stew and agonize over a problem in isolation, which is tantamount to leaving it on an interminable, high-heat spin cycle. Obsessing about the problem causes it to expand to massive proportions, so the problem begins to meld with your identity, inseparable from you. It begins to feel utterly unsolvable. That makes you feel awful, because now it's you who's unsolvable, and ashamed of who you are: a piece of shit who can't solve their own problems. Am I right?

Dreading any contact with that awful, unsolvable

problem, Your Addict will do its damndest to prevent you from asking for help so you can actually deal with the problem. God forbid you should talk about it honestly with anyone. Doing so would mean outing yourself as shameful and unsolvable.

Needless to say, most problems approached in this fashion, including addiction itself, tend to go unsolved.

But hey! Why bother solving problems when Your Addict is ready and waiting with a quick and easy remedy to numb the pain of those problems? That's where your drug comes in, of course. Quick and easy, yes — but with a non-negotiable side of soul-sucking, life-destroying consequences.

So you curse Your Addict, that con artist, who always makes it seem like your drug is the answer to all your problems. You swear you'll never listen to it again. But man, is Your Addict convincing. It's seductive, like a toxic lover. You fall for it, time and time again, going against your better judgment, your values, your intentions, and everything and everyone you love.

Are you convinced yet that Your Addict is the problem? Good. I'll say it again: the first step toward solving a problem is admitting that there is a problem.

The next step, understanding how to solve the problem, will require you to have a basic understanding of how Your Addict came to be, and who it had to kill, maim, or seduce to get where it is today. Basically, Your Addict started out like one of those little capsules that kids put in water. You know, the ones that slowly expand into a giant sponge shaped like a Tyrannosaurus Rex.

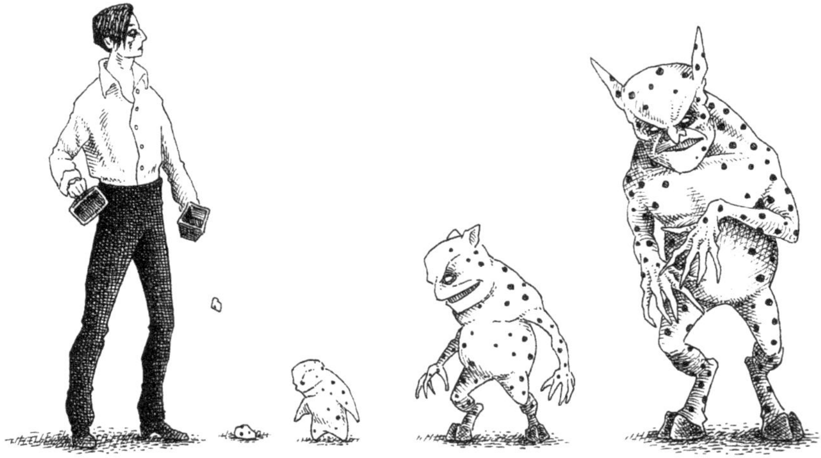

There's no way to get the T. Rex back in the capsule, is there?

That's what happened with you and your drug. You had a taste of it, and it felt good. It enhanced your sense of pleasure, or helped you avoid pain, or both. Then your poor, gullible limbic system — the part of your brain that controls motivation and emotion — sprung into action to re-create that experience, because *man, remember how good that feeling was? Remember how it helped you feel pleasure, and avoid pain?*

From there, Your Addict grew up big and strong. Get ready for a medley of metaphors, because they all apply. Your Addict is like a vacuum, and like all vacuums, it seeks to fill itself. Your Addict is like a tapeworm living inside you, whose appetite keeps getting bigger and bigger. But mostly, Your Addict is a leech in need of a host to supply and protect it.

That's where Your True Self comes in.

CHAPTER 4

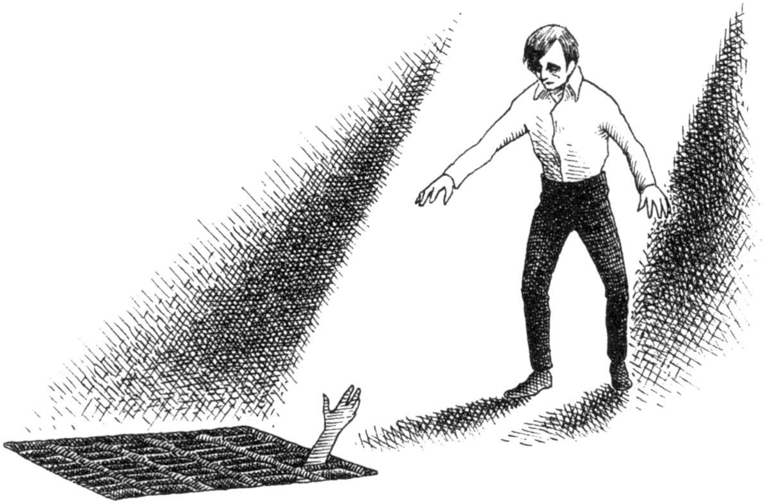

Your True Self... It's in There!

My dear Addict friends, Your True Self is the golden egg nestled deep within you, sparkling and precious. Your True Self contains the best of you, and all your potential. It consists of all the love and light you can bring to your own and others' lives, and all the strengths and capabilities you can offer the world.

I don't care if you've never experienced or acknowledged the beauty of Your True Self. It's there, a brilliant thing that's designed to create, contribute, and connect. Your True Self understands that reaching out to others and having great relationships bring joy and meaning to life. Your True Self wants so much to swim free and strong in the stream of humanity. It wants to grow. It wants to bloom.

Which is another way of saying, Your True Self wants to *love*.

Yes, Your True Self is all about love, my dear Addict friends. As such, it blossoms and flourishes under conditions of love. That's why I plan to spend plenty of time swatting you gently over the head with the truth: that love is both the process and the goal of recovery itself. In this book, you will be learning all about love, which I will refer to by its proper name.

Unconditional Love.

For now, close your eyes and see if you can summon Your True Self by taking a deep, slow breath from the very bottom of your being. Is it protesting like mad in there, banging its fists from underneath the staggering weight of Your Addict? Or do you hear it only faintly, a forlorn voice echoing somewhere within, singing a sad song of loss and longing?

Maybe you don't feel Your True Self at all right now. That's understandable. Over the years, Your Addict may have done a bang-up job of strangling Your True Self into silent submission, all but squelching out that natural-born love and light. But that doesn't mean Your True Self isn't there. I have a hunch, in fact, that Your True Self is the one who picked out this book. It has the will to live, and it knows there's still so much to live for.

That's why, no matter how big and badass Your Addict gets, you still feel the emotional tugging of Your True Self. It still cries out to you pitifully, like an orphaned puppy. More often than not, it gives up and retreats to a corner, paws over its eyes, devastated to bear witness to the destruction Your Addict has wrought. But it still knows exactly what's going on.

You know that inner conflict well. It's called *shame*, and it flares and festers when Your Addict forces Your True Self to betray itself. Your Addict positively thrives on shame, because shame makes you unacceptable to yourself. Shame makes you all the more likely to do whatever it takes to make yourself go away — and along with you, that awful feeling of unacceptability. You'll feed Your Addict like a king, hungering for just those few moments of relief when you can forget how badly you feel about yourself.

But that relief comes at a crushing price: the sure and steady suffocation of Your True Self. It's literally dying for a way out. And I'm here to tell you that there is a way out.

There is a solution.

CHAPTER 5

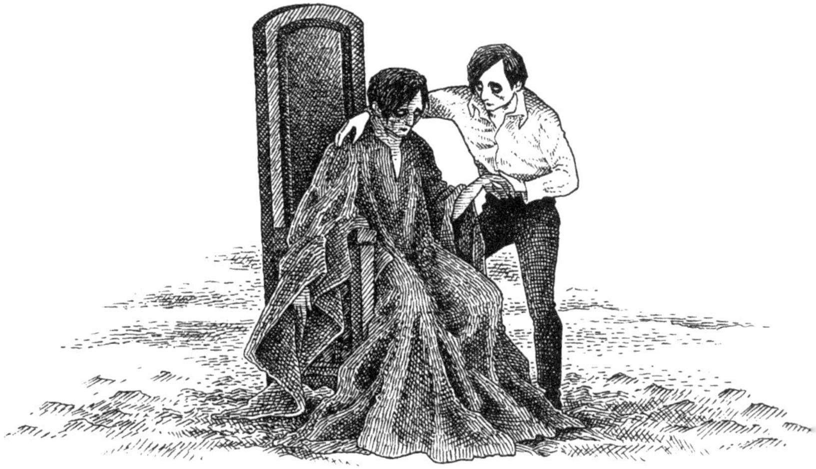

Recovery Is Learning How to Love

Your liberation from Your Addict is a process that comes in two parts. The first part consists of starving and diminishing Your Addict by refusing to feed it your drug. That's called *sobriety*. The other part of the solution is filling the void inside you. The void Your Addict always promised you could fill with your drug — that liar!

Instead of using your drug, you will fill that void with the best possible growing conditions for Your True Self to take root and flourish: love. That's the process called *recovery*. Recovery means learning how to love and take care of Your True Self — and, by extension, learning to love other people, as well as the world around you.

Did you catch the word "process" in there, or should I say it a few more times for emphasis?

Recovery is a process.
Recovery is a process.
Recovery is a process.

That's right; recovery is a process, not an event. Learning to love yourself and the life you're living is a muscle you'll develop with practice. I say "practice," because recovery is something you'll have to get up and decide to do every day until it becomes second nature. (Er, make that your true nature.) That's as opposed to a one-and-done, *poof!* type of transformation — as many people erroneously suppose a three-month stay at an inpatient rehab will be.

Practicing a program of recovery on a daily basis is what will enable you to forge a path of positive growth, even in the midst of life's inevitable pain, problems, and setbacks — which potentially includes relapse.

Likewise, recovery isn't about gritting your teeth and white-knuckling life without your drug. It's about cultivating the good stuff: a sense of peace, freedom, and happiness within you. That's why recovery isn't just about staying sober; it's about making your life meaningful. Love is what gives life meaning and purpose. And in the day to day, love is also what makes Your True Self powerful and resilient.

My dear Addict friends, I'm willing to bet that your biggest challenge in recovery isn't going to be staying sober. Your biggest challenge will be learning to love Your True Self.

The problem is, most addicts have never dared to put the words "self" and "love" together in the same sentence. Instead, we might say something dismissive, like, *self-love just sounds like selfishness or arrogance*. Or maybe, *give me a break, I don't have time for mani-pedis every week in the name of self-love*.

Both of those are deflections, as they miss the point of self-love entirely. Self-love isn't about indulging in spa treatments or thinking you're better than everyone else. Self-love is about accepting yourself unconditionally and empowering yourself to live according to who you are, instead of who you think you should be.

Fostering Unconditional Love for Your True Self is the

only way you'll be able to let go of the shame, denial, and dishonesty that would otherwise continue to sabotage your life in countless ways. Using your drug to escape your feelings may be the most glaring way you've rejected yourself, but I'm sure it's not the only one.

So let's start at the start, by stating the mission of recovery: *learning how to love*. As recovering addicts, we do that by coming to believe in, connect to, and live according to the truth: that love is real, all-powerful, and unconditional. As such, it applies to everyone — us addicts included.

Maybe you're sitting there scratching your head at that. *Love? As the solution to addiction? Is that some kind of joke? Hey lady, don't you know that addiction is a real problem? A freaking disease?*

My dear Addict friends, this is not a book full of medical explanations or complicated psychological interventions for addiction. That's because I didn't write it for doctors and therapists who are trying to treat addicts. I didn't even write it for family members of addicts.

I wrote this book for you.

I wrote this book for all you addicts out there who are just like me. You're aware of the impossibility of living another moment with Your Addict running the show, but you're scared shitless at the prospect of giving up your drug forever. You may feel crazy and ashamed and alone right now, but I can assure you, you are not alone.

That's because My Addict and Your Addict are the same in all the important ways. Your Addict took away your power and fucked up your life, just like mine did. And Your True Self needs Unconditional Love to overpower Your Addict, just like mine does, too.

As fellow human beings (first) and fellow addicts (second), you and I are fundamentally the same. That's why the human solution known as recovery works.

But here's the hard sell for most addicts about recovery. It's not something you learn about once, then go off and do on your own. Recovery is something that Your True Self and My True Self have to do together. There are a lot of reasons for that, as I'll be describing in this book, and the others to come in The Addict's Guide to the Universe series.

But the biggest reason we have to do recovery together is that together-love is ultimately what love is all about.

CHAPTER 6

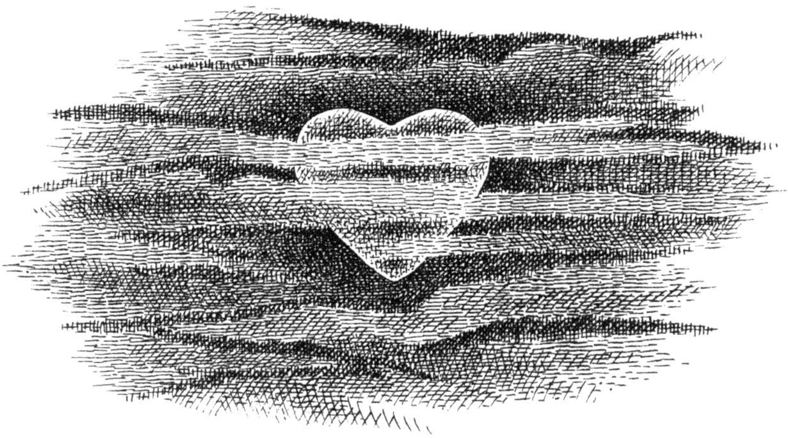

Love Is What You Need

I don't know about you, but I can count at least ten therapists I've had over the past twenty years. I've been prescribed at least fifteen different antidepressants, anti-anxiety medications, and mood stabilizers.

And I've bought so many self-help books, I could start my own lending library specializing exclusively in personal dysfunction.

Books about addiction. Books about recovery. About depression. About anxiety. About codependency. Books about changing my mindset, my habits, my diet, my environment, my relationships, and just about every other facet of my life that the self-help industry could think of.

I've bought and tried and consumed all this stuff with the honorable intention of making myself a happier, healthier person. Some of it helped me achieve a basic level of functioning. Some of it helped me understand myself better. Some of it was just plain entertaining. But none of it helped My True Self get stronger, or weakened My Addict one bit.

In other words, none of it helped me recover.

Yet as I write this today, I'm the happiest and healthiest I've ever been. What changed me wasn't the books. It wasn't the medications. It wasn't even the therapists — not the way I used to lie to them, anyway. The craziest thing is that what's worked for me has been absolutely free, not to mention plentiful. What's worked has had nothing to do with the latest advances in addiction research or psychology. And at this point, I can honestly say that what's working for me doesn't really feel like work at all.

But before I discuss the divine and miraculous solution that's given me the power to free My True Self from the chains of My Addict, I would like to make one request: that you close your eyes for a moment, and visualize your mind as an open door. No locks, no fences, no complicated security codes. Now, leave that door open for the duration of this book, if you will. Even just a crack, if that's all you can manage. Thank you.

Here goes: what keeps me sober, what keeps me healthy, and what keeps me happy today is *love*.

Not watching YouTube videos about love. Not listening to podcasts about love. Not reading about love. Not meditating on it, or taking master classes on it, or even sitting around talking about it. What's worked is actually going out and practicing love — with other people, yes, but with myself, unconditionally.

I can assure you that before I began walking the road of recovery, I didn't know the first thing about love. But I've learned — and I'm still learning. How to accept that I need love. How to ask for love. How to give love. How to receive love. How to appreciate love. How to show myself love. How wonderful real love feels. And above all, how to practice love in my day-to-day life.

You can learn too, my dear Addict friends. That means that you, too, can live a peaceful, free, and happy life, safe from the soul-sucking, shame-inducing clutches of Your Addict. I have all the faith in the world about that.

Now for the bad news.

I wish I could tell you that the people you already have in your life — the people you already know and love and feel more or less comfortable around — are the people who are going to teach you all about love. I wish I could tell you that those are the people who will patiently guide you along the steep and winding learning curve of love as you stumble awkwardly in the dark for a while.

Alas, those are not the people who are going to help you learn how to love.

As a matter of fact, the people who are going to help you learn how to love are a bunch of people you don't know from Adam right now. They're going to be people who don't know what kind of house you live in. Or what you do for a living. Or where you grew up, or who you're married to. Or, God forbid, how much money you make.

Believe me when I tell you that the people who are going to teach you how to love aren't even going to know your last name. And I can assure you that it's going to be much, much better that way. Because none of that stuff is important. Those details would all be one big, unnecessary distraction when it comes to learning how to love unconditionally.

I can also assure you that these people I'm talking about — these strangers — are the people who know you better than you know yourself right now. I'll even venture to say that they know you on a deeper level than some of the people who have known you since birth.

Before I elaborate on these strangers, though, let's talk about the familiar people. Like your friends and family. Or your coworkers. Your neighbors. The one-dimensional faces that make up your social media feeds. I don't mean any offense to those people, because I know they mostly mean well. And many of them do love you. But we both know they can't possibly love all of you.

That's because those people don't know (or don't want to know) about Your Addict.

One of the loneliest things about those people not knowing about Your Addict is that they don't understand the pain it's causing you. They don't understand how powerless you feel to stop using your drug. They don't understand your feelings of despair about your own out-of-control behavior. And the fact that they don't know or understand those things exacerbates your feelings of shame, isolation, and deep, deep loneliness.

Maybe those people don't know or understand Your Addict because you've refused to talk about it. You've denied, debated, or deflected the truth about Your Addict because you don't want to burden them. After all, they might be shocked to learn about the extent of the damage Your Addict has done to your life. They might be frightened. Despondent. Judgmental. Maybe all of the above.

That's not to say that some of them haven't gotten to

know Your Addict for themselves, even without you telling them about it. They may have had direct experience with Your Addict, if only because they live or work or spend the kind of time with you that makes it impossible to hide everything from them, as much as you've pretended you could.

Even so, the people who have seen Your Addict for themselves might be pretty good at pretending, too. They may have turned a blind eye and pretended they weren't seeing it. Or they may have the wrong idea about what it's going to take to overcome Your Addict, pretending that you're capable of freeing yourself on your own. That's why they beg and plead with you to *just stop it, just freaking stop it already, can't you see what this is doing to you? To me? To us?*

Unfortunately, anyone who doesn't know or understand Your Addict can't give you the kind of love that will help you start letting go of your shame, isolation, and loneliness: Unconditional Love. And what you need right now is love that looks straight into the eyes of Your Addict, and refuses to back away out of intimidation or misunderstanding.

You need the kind of love that gets it.

That's why the first step toward connecting to Unconditional Love is being honest about Your Addict with other recovering addicts — the people who are guaranteed to get it. I'll be talking more later on about how that connection works. For now, it's enough to say that the honesty and Unconditional Love you'll be learning to practice in recovery will ultimately allow you to make a peaceful home within Your True Self, in your very real life. It's going to feel more and more natural, as well as necessary, to share Your True Self with an expanding circle of friends and family, and as a loving contributor to the world around you.

Welcome, my beloved Addict friends, to the deeply existential journey that is recovery. Where the only carry-on baggage you need to bring is honesty, open-mindedness, and the willingness to love and live as Your True Self. If there's one seed I want to plant in your heart as we begin to walk this road together, it's a sense of shameless hope in your bright and beautiful future in recovery.

So here's the first thing we're gonna have to do: starve Your Addict — and put Your True Self on an embarrassingly excessive diet of love, love, and even more love.

Unconditional Love.

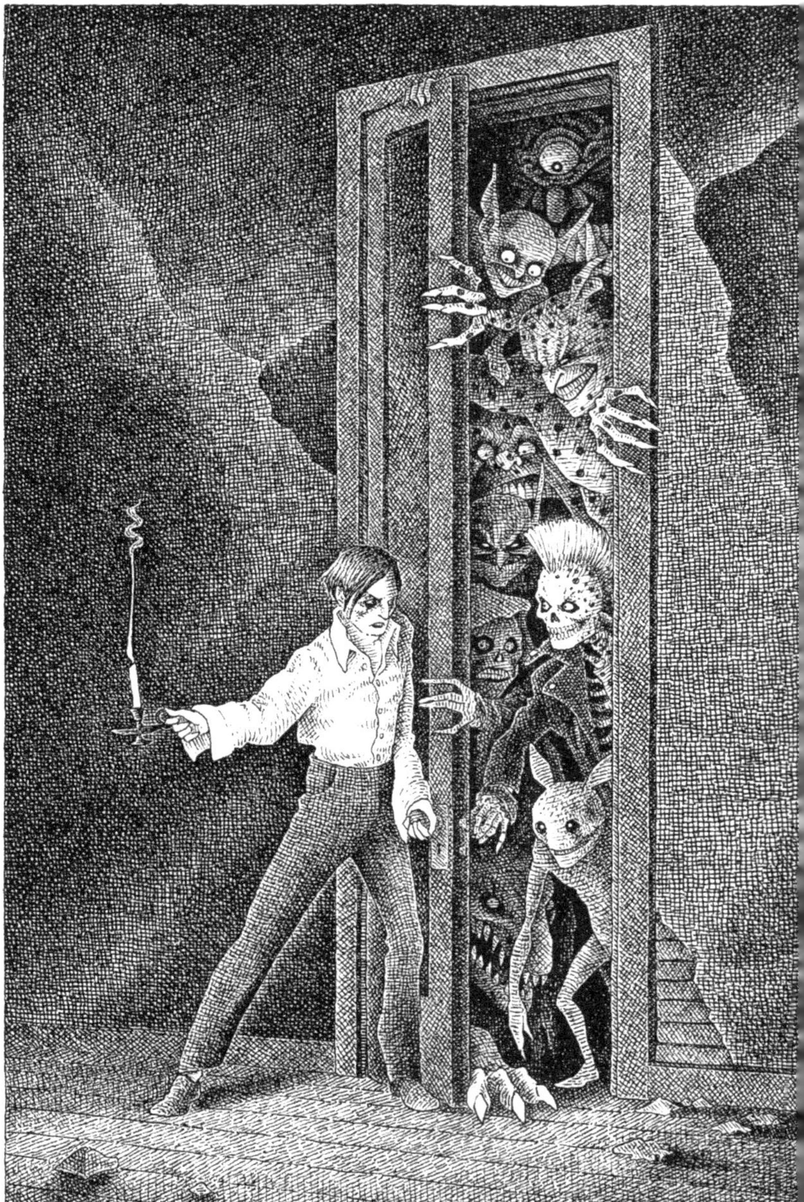

SECTION 2

SOBRIETY

CHAPTER 7

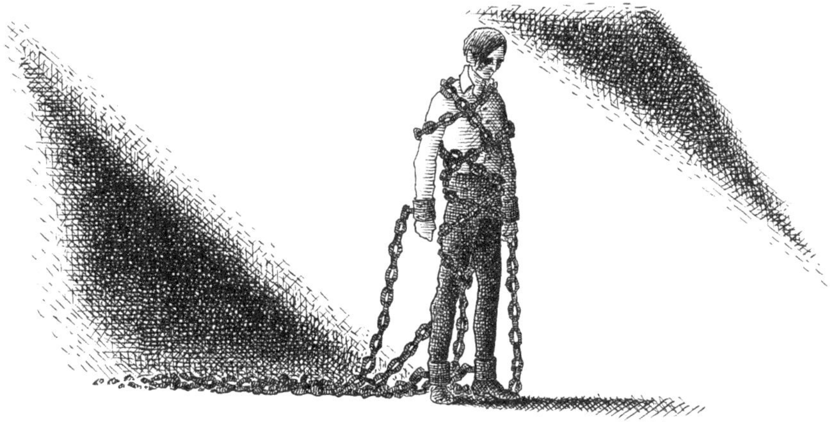

Admitting Powerlessness

My dear Addict friends, let's talk about the word "powerless," shall we? It's a word that's struck fear into the heart of many a would-be recovering addict — so much so, that quite a few run screaming in the opposite direction from recovery.

Here's an example, from a call I got from a potential client. She started off by telling me how grateful she was to have found a therapist who specialized in recovery. Then she went on to describe the mounting problems in her life that prompted her call.

The husband whose guts she hated, because he was never home. The stepdaughter who hated her guts. The career that seemed stuck in neutral. The friends who had abandoned her in her time of need. And the many days spent languishing in a grimy puddle of remorse and regret over how many bottles of wine she had consumed the night before.

After that, she inquired about my approach to treatment. "Are you one of those all-or-nothing therapists?" she asked, before daring to utter the dirtiest word in the English language to an addict who's still using. "Are you going to tell me to get... *sober*?"

"That decision will always be up to you," I said. "My job is to try to help people move beyond the crazy, painful struggle of trying to control what can't be controlled, so they have the freedom to focus on their life again."

I went on to explain that for the vast majority of recovering people, trying to have *just one drink* (or the equivalent of another drug) will fling open the doors to powerlessness again, often sooner rather than later.

I don't know if she heard much of what I said after the word "powerlessness," though. Because she sure was in a hurry to get off the phone after that.

"Oh, I don't think I'm powerless over alcohol," she said, before telling me that she would keep looking for a therapist who wouldn't try to take alcohol away from her. "I just want to learn to control my emotions, so I don't feel like I want to drink so much."

After she hung up, I felt like banging my head against a wall. *That's putting the cart before the horse!* I wanted to shout into the phone she was no longer on the other end of. How could she fail to see how her out-of-control unhappiness was connected to her out-of-control alcohol use?

But I do know how that happens: denial.

I remember how hard it was for me, for so many years, to connect the dots between my addictions and my unhappiness. I was terrified of letting go of drugs and alcohol, because substances seemed like the only way to find relief and release from the weight of my feelings. If those were taken away from me, it stood to reason that I would have no power whatsoever to help myself feel better.

That's why I understand how impossible, how counterintuitive, and how terrifying the prospect is of giving up the security blanket that is your drug — especially in the midst of your unhappiness. It's human nature to try to protect ourselves from the truth, when that truth has terrifying implications. That's why so many addicts spend so long in denial about their powerlessness before the bottom falls out on their lives, and they can't ignore the truth a minute longer.

So this is what I'd say to an addict struggling to come to terms with their powerlessness — and along with that, the prospect of sobriety as the inevitable remedy.

Admitting powerlessness over your drug doesn't make you a weak person.

It doesn't make you a failure, either. It doesn't mean you will never have fun again. And it doesn't mean you will lose your power to comfort yourself in the face of difficult feelings. Admitting powerlessness is simply one of the first steps you'll have to take to start walking the road of recovery.

This is the road that grants you the power to break every limitation you've ever put upon yourself, or that others have put upon you. This is the road that grants you the power to overcome the fears and untangle the lies that have prevented you from living a peaceful, free, and happy life as Your True Self.

Unlike the collaborative, cooperative, and interdependent nature of nearly everything else you'll do in recovery, though, admitting powerlessness is a step you'll have to take on your own. I mean that in the sense that the truth of it has to come from you, and you alone. Ultimately, I can't tell anyone else that they're powerless, and have it mean anything constructive.

That's why I'm here to hold your hand, my dear Addict friends, as I gently guide you along the road of truth. The road of truth is the road of love, which is the only real security, and the only real release, from powerlessness. And I don't just mean powerlessness over your drug. I mean powerlessness over your feelings, your thoughts, your behavior, and the direction of your life itself.

Speaking of truth, I'd like to reiterate that admitting powerlessness over your drug is not a moral failing. It has nothing to do with the strength of your character, or of your inherent deficiency as a person. Neither is it an indication of how uncool you are, because you can't control your drug the way other people seem to be able to.

Powerlessness over your drug just is.

Researchers have pointed to a whole host of factors that contribute to addiction, trying to answer the question of why some people progressively lose control over a certain drug or behavior, and others don't. Some research points to genetics, or to social conditioning, or to trauma, or to personality. Some research points to a combination of them all.

The *why?* question may be an interesting one, but it's only slightly more helpful to your recovery than trying to answer the shame and blame-laced question of *why me?* Do you need to know how electricity works in order to flip on a light switch? Do you need to understand the laws of physics to restrain yourself from jumping off a building?

Besides, there will be plenty of time to dig into the roots of your addictive personality — i.e., Your Addict — once you're sober. We can't put the cart before the horse. It's only when you take away your drug, whose function was to numb or transform you, that you'll have access to the feelings and facts that will help you make sense of how your emotional and behavioral patterns came to be.

Right now, *why?* won't move you forward, nor will raging against the injustice of your condition. Accepting the truth about your powerlessness will.

Let's look at a few examples of what everyday powerlessness looks like for an addict. Perhaps you can relate to these instances of Your Addict robbing Your True Self of its rightful position as the CEO of your life.

- Powerlessness is letting Your Addict drive the car when your kids are in the backseat.
- Powerlessness is somehow being in the wrong place at the wrong time, for each and every one of your DUIs.
- Powerlessness is bruises from accidents you don't remember.
- Powerlessness is spending money you don't have on something you don't need.
- Powerlessness is waking up wracked with shame about what you did last night — or not remembering last night at all.
- Powerlessness is losing things — like jobs, marriages, hobbies, or good friends — that you'd have much preferred to keep.

- Powerlessness is breaking up with Your Addict every single night, then getting back together with it the very next day.
- Powerlessness is hating Your Addict's guts even as you're right there with it, feeding it and choosing it above everything else.
- Powerlessness is failing to control your use of your drug every time you do use it, even though you swore to yourself that you could control it, you would control it. *Just this time, just one more time.*

Your True Self may have 563 excellent reasons to tell Your Addict to take a hike, and only one bullshit excuse to use your drug: *because I want it!* Powerlessness is that one impulsive thought hijacking all your powers of reason, at exactly the wrong moment.

Please note that you didn't hear "living under a bridge squatting on a dirty mattress and clutching a paper bag from the package store" in any of these examples of powerlessness. That's because there are an awful lot of well-dressed professionals with nice houses and good families who are suffering under the weight of unacknowledged powerlessness.

My dear Addict friends, no matter who you are or what you look like, addiction always manifests as powerlessness: not having the power to control your use of your drug. So simple, yet so baffling. So insane.

Your Addict has taken away your power, and left you powerless over your drug.

Yet even as the rats are fleeing Your Addict's sinking ship, you relish the illusory comfort that comes from trying, over and over, to prove that you are more powerful than your drug. You tell yourself that you'll only use it on weekends or Wednesdays; you'll drink beer but not booze; you'll snort but not shoot up; you'll restrict yourself to betting on basketball instead of going to the casino.

But no. No, you can't control it. As long as you're engaging with your drug, it's not a question of *if*, but *when* your use of your drug will deposit you squarely in a steaming pile of powerlessness again. I hate to break it to you, but all that time you've spent negotiating with your drug, you've just been feeding Your Addict and helping it grow stronger.

It's true. The more you try to control your drug, the more powerless you become. That's why the foundation of recovery is surrendering your futile bid for power and control. The battle is fixed, and you can't win. Accept it, so you don't waste any more time or drag yourself down fighting.

Take heart, my dear Addict friends, that accepting your powerlessness doesn't mean defeat. It means you're joining forces with the all-powerful ally that is *truth*. And there's nothing more true than the fact that the truth will set you free. Unconditional Love will see to it.

CHAPTER 8

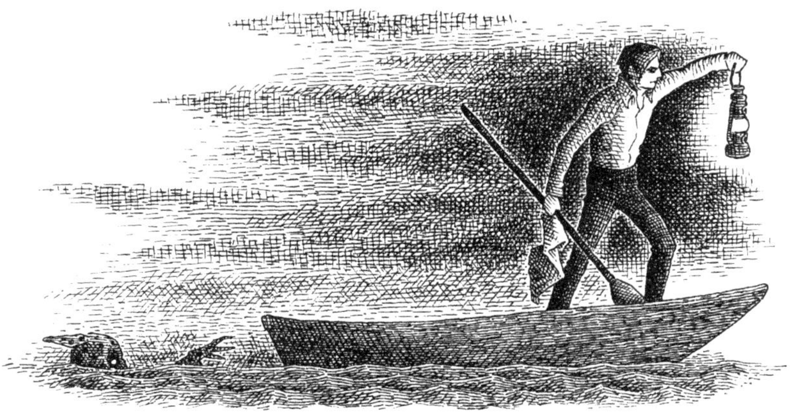

Sobriety Is a Process

My dear Addict friends, when it comes to what it takes to live in recovery, there is no issue more contentious, or fraught with anxiety — or, dare I say, gray and murky — than that of sobriety.

So for those of you just starting out on this road — and even for some who have been walking it for a while — it's essential to talk about what sobriety means. What practicing sobriety entails. How necessary sobriety is, and to what extent. And then there's the big kahuna of sobriety questions, about the possibility for eventual reunification with your drug.

The least reassuring (but also the truest) thing I can tell you right off the bat is that *sobriety* is a relative term. Meaning, the answers to those questions will vary considerably from person to person.

Please hear me when I say that just like recovery itself, sobriety is a process, not an event, for most recovering addicts. It often takes a great deal of trial and error, along with plenty of honest self-reflection and open dialogue along the way, to determine what application of sobriety you will need to practice in order to live a peaceful, free, and happy life.

My own sobriety was just such a process. While I would consider marijuana to be My Addict's ride-or-die drug of choice, I have a history of abusing pretty much every substance I could get my hands on, going all the way back to my teens. If it had the potential to change my mood or obliterate my consciousness, My Addict would rise up like a great big greedy beast, demanding more and more of it — to hell with the consequences.

My Addict was a big part of my life from the start, and I followed its lead for more than fifteen years. After that, my own sobriety unfolded over a ten-year period. I got sober from cocaine, Ecstasy, and prescription stimulants more than a decade before I stopped using weed. In between, I got sober from alcohol and benzodiazepine meds. I now practice sobriety from them all.

But at no time during that ten-year process could you have forced me, shamed me, or tried to talk me into quitting any one of those substances one single second before I actually did. I wasn't ready until I was ready, to use one of the truest truisms of recovery. My sobriety has been a process of gradual awareness and acceptance that I cannot enjoy a life of peace, freedom, and happiness if I use any of those substances. Believe me, I've tried to finagle them every which way, and I can't.

That's just me, though. And I have to be careful not to apply the same *I know what's best for you!* sobriety logic to everyone who comes to me for help with an addictive disorder. Because for some recovering people, the full-scale sobriety standard is either just not happening, or it doesn't seem to be a prerequisite for them to enjoy the freedoms of recovery.

Regardless of the reason, I don't believe that anyone should be shamed or coerced into adhering to a standard of sobriety that they aren't ready for, or that doesn't make sense to them. If complete sobriety from all substances is what you authentically need and want, that's terrific. If not, then it's critical to begin your recovery by exploring your willingness to get sober from the drug(s) you are clearly powerless over — the source of your out-of-control behavior, declining health, and emotional distress.

I recognize that there are plenty of people in the world of recovery (which includes both recovering addicts and the professionals who treat them) who believe that an addict is an addict is an addict, and that any addict who wants to recover needs to abstain from every potentially addictive substance, lest he or she risk becoming addicted to whatever could fill the void left behind by their drug of choice. To them, sobriety means no more alcohol or potentially addictive drugs — forever. (One day at a time, of course.)

I once saw a documentary about marijuana addiction where one of the addicts interviewed said, "If you put me on the moon without any weed around, I'd be smoking moon rocks in no time." A good number of us addicts are simply wired that way. If there's an accessible emergency exit that allows us to escape ourselves, we'll head that way instinctively, no matter how well things are going otherwise.

I have a problem, though, when the total-sobriety people start condemning other recovering addicts who aren't doing the same. Because shaming and peer pressure are such effective motivators for positive change… not.

Besides, what I've observed is that even such an unequivocal approach to sobriety isn't a hard and fast solution guaranteeing peace, freedom, and happiness.

What if a recovering alcoholic is successful at abstaining from all addictive drugs, but he obsessively pursues a series of intense, short-term relationships — the inevitable failure of which sends him into frequent spirals of despair and self-loathing? Such a person wouldn't be able to reap the benefits of recovery, as long as he's engaging in such self-destructive behavior.

Unfortunately, I've seen many recovering addicts suffer when they turn a blind eye to the impact of their dubious extracurricular activities, whether that's compulsive sex, gambling, anger, cigarette smoking, binge eating, video gaming, or workaholism. It can be all too easy to fall into denial about the damage Your Addict continues to inflict, as long as you're busy patting yourself on the back from a lofty tower of chemical sobriety.

Conversely, I've worked with recovering alcoholics who use cannabis edibles before bed without any symptoms of abusing them. I've worked with recovering sex addicts who have a glass of wine with dinner, but don't think twice about alcohol otherwise. I've worked with recovering drug addicts who can put bets on the Super Bowl, or buy the occasional scratch-off ticket, and not get sucked into a gambling addiction.

Who am I to tell these people that they're doing recovery wrong, if they're not experiencing any emotional or behavioral distress as a result of those behaviors? Not that it would matter, even if I did raise an eyebrow. Growth is best facilitated when we can recognize and accept the truth about ourselves — not when other people try to tell us who we are, or what we need to do.

That said, it's entirely possible that behaviors that have historically been non-problematic for you may become problematic. Hence, the trial and error aspect of many recovering addicts' sobriety. Please take heart, though, that falling into another form of addictive behavior doesn't have to spell disaster, or be an ominous indication of your future in recovery.

Instead, I would urge you to regard any slips back into powerlessness as critical information about what doesn't work for you anymore. The most important thing is your capacity to admit that there's a problem, followed by your willingness to address it. Both of those skills will come with time, as you scale the learning curve of honesty and self-reflection that are integral to recovery.

In the big picture, sobriety is about having our eyes wide open to the behaviors and circumstances that are harmful to us, and becoming willing to let those go when we accept that truth.

CHAPTER 9

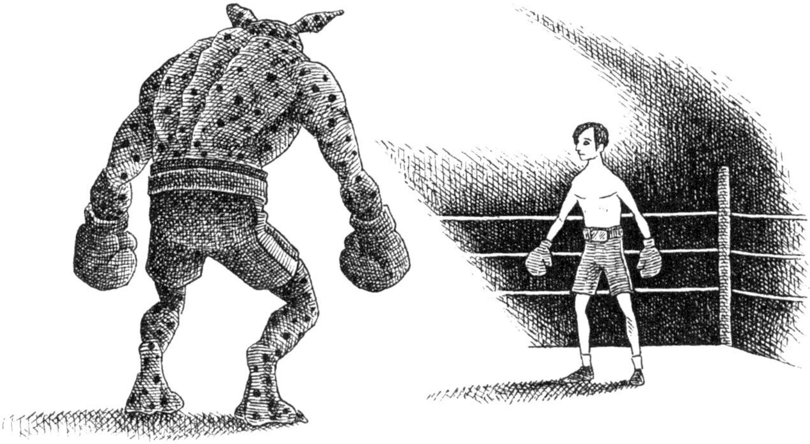

Willpower and Control

There are plenty of sober addicts out there who aren't in recovery. Many of them are just gritting their teeth instead of using their drug. They may be so ashamed of having an addiction that their hearts and minds are closed to asking for help from other recovering addicts — the people uniquely capable of helping them learn how to love.

These are people who shun the idea of recovery meetings, and perhaps professional therapy as well. They regard their independence and self-sufficiency as a badge of honor.

In my experience, such people are generally miserable in sobriety. They live every day peering into the dark void left behind by their drug, but are afraid to look

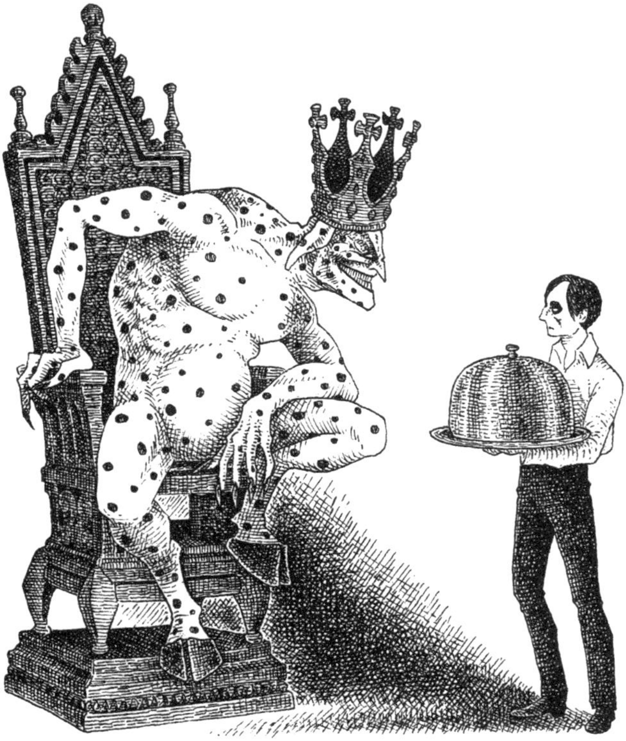

beyond themselves and venture into the unknown to fill it. They tell themselves that all they need to stay sober is their own willpower. These people are closed circuits, relying only on themselves to *be strong!* and stay away from their drug.

But what a life that would be!

Picture a boxing ring in which Your Addict and your own unsteady willpower are going head-to-head indefinitely, with nothing and no one to help back you up. No relief, no comfort, no sense of security. At worst, that fight would be utterly unsustainable, and you'd wind up flat on the mat while Your Addict did a victory dance around your lifeless body. At best, that fight would be exhausting and demoralizing — day in and day out.

Because even if your willpower could stave off your drug for a while, the tragedy of relying on willpower alone is that you would be spending your days and nights fighting Your Addict, instead of loving Your True Self.

It doesn't have to be that way.

I understand that your future as a sober person in recovery isn't just unknown territory; it's a non-linear and non-quantifiable process. That terrifies the control freak that lies at the heart of Your Addict, that beast who insists on monopolizing your time, energy, attention, and resources to satisfy its black hole of an appetite.

So here's the bad news. There's so much about getting sober that involves letting go of all the control you'd love to have, but never had much of anyway. The classic example of this is the control you've tried to exert over your drug. I know, I know, you'd love to still be able to use your drug on Saturday nights, and perhaps the occasional Thursday evening, too, and of course at social gatherings where everyone else is under the influence of it, and let's throw in your brother's wedding you'll be attending in six months for good measure.

But, um, no. Remember? That's why you're here. You're powerless — meaning, you don't control your drug. Your drug controls you.

Another example of the control we'd love to have (but don't really) is determining for ourselves what it's going to take to get and keep us sober. Examples: *I don't do Twelve Step meetings*, or, *I hate group therapy*, or, *I don't want to talk about my feelings*, or, *I still need to work sixty hours a week and stay in my miserable relationship after I get sober.*

I respect your desires, my dear Addict friends, but as an addiction therapist and your overall recovery fairy, please know that it comes from a place of deep love when I respond to your persistent bids for control with a smarmy remark like, *since when did you know best?*

There's even a recovery cliché that sums it up: *my own best thinking got me here.*

Which is why it's time to surrender control to the benevolent forces of recovery.

CHAPTER 10

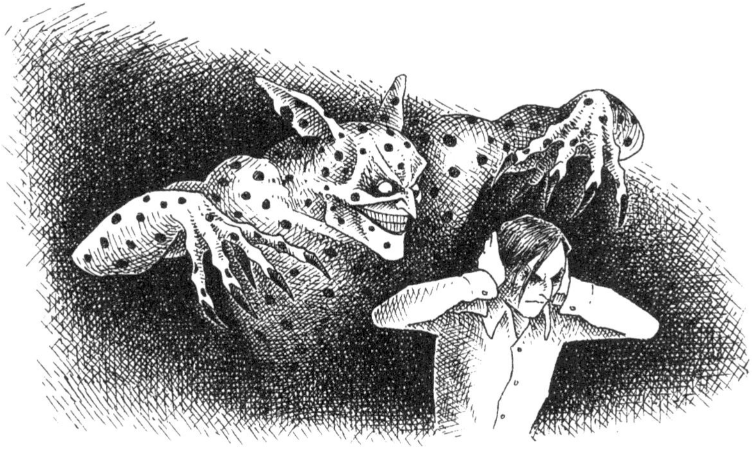

Honest Connection Is the Best Protection

Sobriety is the most fundamental level of honesty for a recovering addict. Call it self-honesty, if you will. That's because sobriety means existing with your unaltered truth, without your drug to hide you from yourself. Sobriety is about *being yourself*, in the most literal sense of the term.

At least initially, though, sobriety also means tolerating the noisy presence of Your Addict. Determined not to go down without a fight, it will rebel furiously against this honesty by trying to get you to go back to your drug. Even as Your Addict slings a barrage of intolerable feelings at you, along with a thousand and one tantalizing thoughts about using your drug, you must not revert to covering up those thoughts and feelings by actually using your drug.

I will warn you that in your first days, weeks, and months of sobriety, those thoughts and feelings might seem unbearable. They might make you feel like you want to crawl out of your own skin. This is not your cue to repress those feelings by running back to your drug, however. Doing so would cause Your Addict to rub its claws together in delight, salivating over how well its excrement-slinging campaign worked to feed its greedy appetite.

Welcome back to the darkness! Your Addict would crow. *Now let's eat! Shall I seat you right down this dark little alley, at your usual shit-smeared table for one?*

No, those unbearable feelings are your cue to release those unbearable feelings by being honest about them. Rather than running for dark cover, you must turn those feelings over to the light by connecting to the people who will give you a boost of powerful Unconditional Love in return — instead of using your drug, which comes laced with crippling shame and a bottomless need for more.

The people you most need to be honest with about those feelings are the strangers I talked about earlier: your fellow recovering addicts. Otherwise known as the people uniquely capable of giving you the Unconditional Love you need right now to stay sober and learn to love Your True Self.

Your fellow recovering addicts will be accepting of what you reveal when you shine the light of honesty on all your ugly, unbearable thoughts and feelings. After all, they've experienced those themselves. They will also express hope for Your True Self in a way that no non-recovering, non-addict could.

I have a feeling you may already know where to find these recovering addicts, but in case you don't, I'll clue you in.

I'll start with the free, community-based Twelve Step fellowships that meet every day, both in person and online, every hour, and in every time zone, all over the world. The granddaddy of those is Alcoholics Anonymous, which was founded back in the 1930s by a couple of recovering alcoholics who found they could successfully stay sober by providing support to each other. They recognized that this mutual support was a power greater than their own individual resources of willpower, which had always proved inadequate when it came to sobriety.

By facilitating regular meetings of recovering alcoholics, who in turn carried that message of mutual support to an ever-expanding network of other alcoholics in need, the A.A. fellowship grew exponentially over the decades that followed. As of 2020, its size was estimated at two million members worldwide, though the challenge of collecting accurate statistics on an anonymous, non-hierarchical, loosely organized fellowship should be noted.

That network of support has expanded to address much more than alcoholism. Today, there are Twelve Step fellowships that help addicts recover from just about every substance and addictive behavior out there, from marijuana to cocaine to gambling to sex to codependency to overeating, and plenty more. What that means is that there are recovering addicts who are powerless over your drug, too. They're ready to accept you, to help you, to listen to you, and to share their own stories of addiction and recovery.

Besides Twelve Step, there are other free, community-based, mutual support recovery fellowships, such as SMART Recovery, LifeRing, and Women for Sobriety. I have done my best to compile a list of these, along with their contact information, in the Resources section here. Please note that I cannot vouch for how those programs work, since my personal and professional experience has been limited to various Twelve Step fellowships, both the secular and faith-based variety.

Bottom line: I am not a stickler about which recovery fellowship my dear Addict friends connect to, as long as it involves the opportunity to meet regularly and talk honestly with other recovering addicts.

Even before you're ready to get sober, or to accept the truth about your powerlessness over your drug, attending these meetings is a terrific way to get started on the road of recovery. Getting honest with other recovering addicts about what you're struggling with is a powerful step toward helping yourself out of that struggle. Or, if you're not comfortable opening up just yet, you can listen with an open mind to their honesty.

Of course, the last thing Your Addict wants is for you to be honest about what you're struggling with. How dare you open your eyes and ears to anything beyond the echo chamber of its odious demands upon you! How dare you foster hope that you could learn to live and love yourself without your drug!

To protect itself, Your Addict will feed you a thousand and one reasons why you're not one of *those people*. It will object that you're too busy for meetings, or too bored, or too addicted, or not addicted enough, or that they believe in things you'll never believe in, or that you won't be able to relate in any number of other ways.

Blah, blah, blah. Don't be fooled into taking any of those excuses seriously. They're defensive tactics, designed to prevent you from doing anything that would threaten

Your Addict's chokehold of power and control over you.

As I've said, the people you already know and love may also love you unconditionally, but the fact that they haven't experienced what you're going through will always be a barrier to you believing in, and therefore receiving, their Unconditional Love. You may sense that those people, however loving they are, are full of fear for you. And more fear is the last thing you need right now. You've got plenty of your own, without theirs adding to your stress.

Speaking of fear, I understand that the prospect of being honest with other people about your feelings can be even more terrifying than the brutal self-honesty of practicing sobriety. Honesty with others means allowing them to bear witness to all your naturally occurring fear, shame, and insanity. As if allowing yourself to bear witness to those, sober, wasn't scary enough, right?

Fear not, my dear Addict friends, because the act of unloading your honest baggage with other recovering addicts will be rewarded with a lovely, liberating feeling you will come to know as *relief*. Get used to it. In fact, go ahead and rub it all over your tired, aching, Addict-riddled soul. Relief is another side effect of Unconditional Love, and the good news is that you can give it to yourself, any time you're willing to unburden yourself by exposing your painful thoughts and feelings to the light.

Recovery represents Unconditional Love for Your True Self, for the way it consists of the day-to-day action of telling your truth. That's why sobriety — the foundation of recovery — is about removing the substances and behaviors that are hiding you from yourself. Once you get sober, you get access to your truth again.

But sobriety will be too painful and tenuous to maintain, at least at first, without regular, honest connection with other recovering addicts. Continually pushing yourself to connect to that source of Unconditional Love, by telling your truth and receiving acceptance and hope in return, is what will allow you to start healing what's been hidden and hurting inside you.

CHAPTER 11

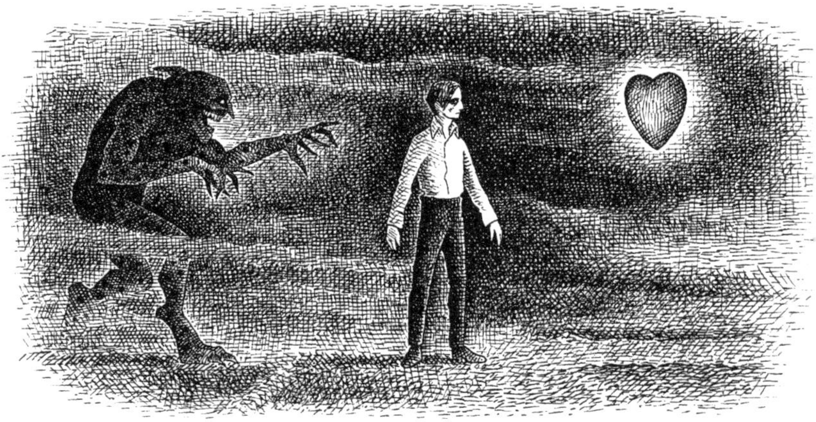

Deciding to Be Sober... Right Now

My dear Addict friends, the road of recovery is paved with a deluge of daily decisions. *Should I make my bed? Should I go to that work party? Should I take the long way home so I don't have to pass the liquor store?*

Of course, life presents you with all the same choices, whether you're in recovery or not. But there's one critical difference that makes all the difference. When Your Addict is the one doing the deciding, *you* aren't making any decisions at all.

See, every time you deflect the problem, or minimize your drug's impact on you, or engage in a futile bid for control over your drug, Your Addict claps its hands together in delight, because that means you're looking the other way. Like a sugar-crazed kid with a distracted mom, it gets to reach its grubby little hand into the cookie jar just that much deeper, and for that much longer.

Thank God your head is no longer stuck in the sandbox of denial! Now you understand that your biggest problem is Your Addict, and that the way you allow its power over you to expand is by feeding it your drug.

As interminably powerless as you may be over your drug, though, the good news is that you don't have to let Your Addict do your deciding for you any longer. Your biggest step toward taking back your power will be the day you decide to stop feeding Your Addict, in an unequivocal mass starvation.

I'm talking about the day that marks your massive decision to make just one decision: the decision to be sober from your drug, *right now*.

Though I hope you will come to celebrate that day as your sobriety birthday, I want to point out that the decision to initiate the unequivocal mass starvation of Your Addict is not of the one-and-done variety. Especially in the first year or two of recovery, sobriety has to be a decision you make one day at a time. It's simply too overwhelming, too confounding, and too terrifying, otherwise.

Sometimes, sobriety has to be a minute-by-minute, or even a second-by-second, decision.

In that sense, your decision to be sober isn't one single decision at all, but a series of many successive decisions that will amount to building up Your True Self's power, and diminishing Your Addict's. But I don't want to overwhelm you, because the only decision you have to be concerned with right now concerns the *right now*.

What's that you're saying, my dear Addict friend? That you're not ready to make the decision to be sober, *right now*?

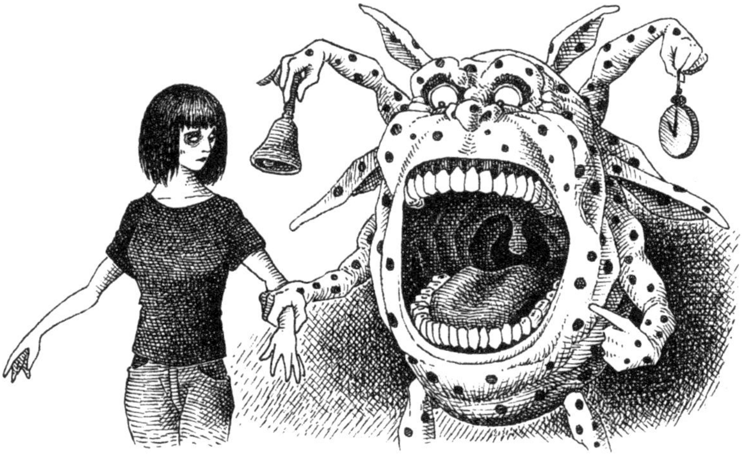

If that's the case, then I thank you for your honesty. Feeling afraid to live without your drug is completely normal. We're addicts, after all. Being emotionally, physically, and psychologically dependent on our drug is what we do! I can assure you, though, that being honest about where you are, wherever you are, is the first step toward actually getting sober — next to admitting powerlessness, which is also an act of brutal honesty.

So if you don't feel ready to be sober, you can still start facing your fears by being honest about them with the kind of people who get it. Just don't kid yourself that fear isn't the issue. Don't delude yourself that you have good reasons for choosing to wait until your birthday to get sober. Or until the day after the Fourth of July. Or until New Year's Day, that ol' *I'm gonna be sober this year, I swear!* standby.

Picking a date well into the future can only mean one thing: that fear is plunking you back down in the sandbox of denial, which is exactly where Your Addict wants you.

So screw the idea of picking a sobriety date. Start with *right now.*

First, though, a critical note. If your drug is alcohol, or benzodiazepine meds, or opioids (whether in the form of prescription pain medication or heroin), your first step toward sobriety must be a visit to a medical professional. Depending on the substance, the withdrawal symptoms from those drugs aren't just uncomfortable, they can cause seizures, strokes, severe dehydration, or even death if not medically monitored.

You will need a medical professional to evaluate your current severity of use, as well as your history of past withdrawal symptoms, to determine whether it's safe to stop using your drug on your own. If not, you may need to undergo a supervised detoxification and withdrawal process, which can range anywhere from a few days to a few weeks.

That said, many of you will be able to get started on the road of recovery without going to an inpatient detox or rehabilitation program. It's my clinical experience that the majority of addicts who want to get sober do not require medical supervision during their withdrawal process. But do yourself a big favor, and check with your doctor first.

I'll remind you, though, that no one can do recovery by themselves. Going it alone is, by definition, not recovery. Remember, recovery is the process of learning to love Your True Self that recovering addicts help each other practice — together. And nowhere is that more true than when it comes to your early days of getting sober.

I say that because for most of us addicts, making the decision to be sober from our drug feels like taking a flying leap of faith off a tall building.

Where will I land? Will I be okay? What will protect me from my feelings and my problems when I don't have my drug anymore?

You will need people who will surround you with a safety net of love and support in the midst of that flying leap. You will need people who can help you identify and endure the withdrawal symptoms you may experience as a result of not using your drug. You will need a lot of reassurance that you're doing the right thing, as well as reminders that the alternative to sobriety — resorting back to powerlessness — is no alternative at all.

You will also need the hope these people will help you cultivate that you, too, can be sober, and that there's a great life in store for you beyond your drug.

While it's true that no one can decide to be sober for you, getting support from others is ultimately what will help you stay sober through all those *right now* moments. Especially on the days when fear threatens to overtake you, and you feel like you're still in the midst of that flying leap off a tall building.

What about all the unknown days stretched ahead of me? you'll think, anxiously. *Will I be able to stay sober through all of those, too?*

And then you'll remember: you are not in free fall. You are on solid ground, as long as you connect to the power of Unconditional Love you need to stay sober — *right now*.

CHAPTER 12

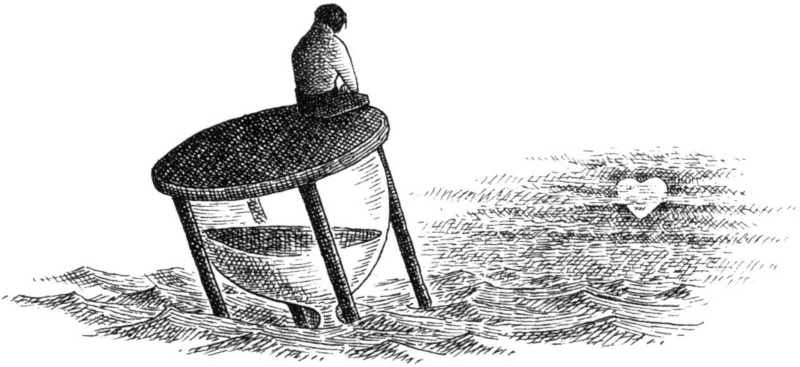

The Craving Will Pass

Okay, I'm about to give you the sagest relapse prevention advice you don't have to spend $10,000 on professional addiction treatment to hear.

The craving will pass, whether you act on it or not.

I'm not sure where I first heard that bit of wisdom. It might have come from my own addiction therapist. Every time I've repeated it to my clients, they've come back and reported how shockingly true, and shockingly helpful, it turned out to be. How repeating it over and over to themselves gave them the faith they needed to not use their drug.

Because the thing about being in the midst of a craving for your drug is that it feels intolerably interminable. You feel like you might combust if you don't get it, or worse, like you'll be stuck in some intensely itchy craving purgatory — forever. To hear a voice of reason telling you, *fear not, dear child, this too shall pass* is often just what you need. It can be the saving grace that allows you to stick out that craving for five more minutes, or even five more hours, until it abates.

The craving will pass, whether you act on it or not is reassuring in a way that another popular get-through-the-craving expression, *you can always use tomorrow*, doesn't quite pull off. Let's face it, a lot of us would jump at the chance to use tomorrow, and we'd spend the rest of today in obsessive anticipation. That's the kind of promise an addict simply doesn't forget.

Even when you're willing to take the leap of faith of actually believing that *the craving will pass, whether you act on it or not*, it still begs one critical question.

What in the hell are you supposed to do until the craving does pass?

SOBER breathing is a relapse prevention exercise I learned about back when I was a rookie addiction therapist, trying to help people on probation stop smoking weed so they could pass their drug tests. "SOBER" is an acronym that can help you remember the five parts of the exercise.

The S in SOBER stands for *stop*. Because when you find yourself starting to think those lovey-dovey thoughts about getting back together with Your Addict, the first thing you need to do is stop right there. Get yourself out of automatic addict pilot mode by ceasing all activity you can, both physical and mental. The purpose of intentional stopping is to interrupt the domino effect of fantasies, excuses, and behaviors that threaten to drive you directly to using.

The O in SOBER stands for *observe*. Now that you're still, take a good look within yourself. Ask yourself what you're feeling and how you're experiencing it. It's a craving, yes, but where do you feel it in your body? Your head? Your chest? Is it in the tightness of your muscles? Observing your discomfort in a non-judgmental way will help you escape the claustrophobia of your craving. Another benefit of getting an objective perspective on what you're feeling is that it helps diminish the delusion that you'll die if you don't satisfy the craving. You won't. That's just Your Addict messing with you again.

The B in SOBER stands for *breathe*. After you've stopped and surveyed yourself, see if you can begin to center yourself on your breath. Take some deep inhales from the bottom of your belly for at least three seconds, then take equal time on your exhale, doing your best to concentrate on the rhythmic movement of your breath. Besides receiving the physiological benefits of more oxygen flowing to your brain, using your mental energy to focus on your breath can distract you from the craving itself. Anything is better than giving your attention to the craving, which only expands its power over you.

Speaking of, the E in SOBER stands for *expand*. You've been focusing on your breath, but now try to expand your attention to your body as a whole, visualizing all the sensations you're experiencing, from your head down to your toes. This is where I find it helpful to start thinking of my body as an ornate temple. Don't laugh! There's something about picturing it as an amazingly intricate and complex system of functioning that tends to lessen the appeal of jacking it up with toxic substances and behaviors.

Finally, the R in SOBER stands for *respond*. Now that you've exercised control over your movement, your breath, your mind, and your body, it can be a good time to get back into your head to consider the range of choices you have at this moment. Surprisingly, there are about a zillion not-so-bad things you can do instead of using your drug. *I could take a walk! Call a friend! Order a pizza! Watch* 'Alien' *again!* As long as it diverts you from your drug, it's fair game.

In the big picture, the best plan for how to wait out a craving is to very intentionally stop what you're doing, and very intentionally take a different path. Bear in mind, though, that your willingness to even bother to wait is contingent upon one thing: faith.

But not blind faith — we're talking about faith in the truth. Namely, that *the craving will pass, whether you act on it or not.*

So ask yourself: which side do you want to be on, when the storm blows over?

CHAPTER 13

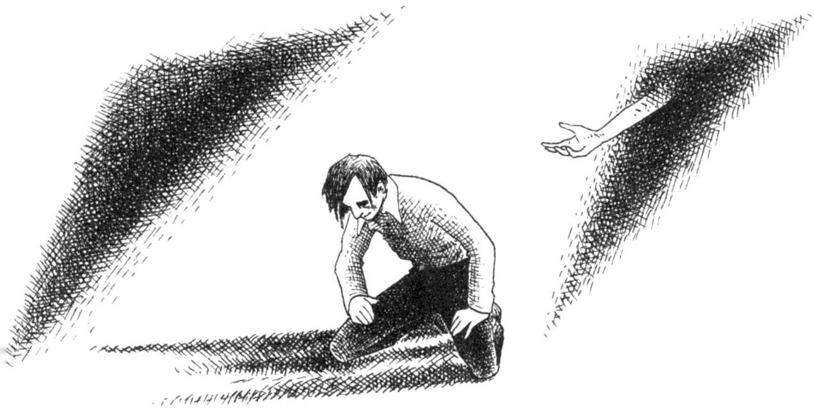

Rebounding From Relapse

Speaking of faith, here's what I consider to be a super helpful way to start getting back on your feet, in case you do relapse on your drug — whether that relapse happens after three years of sobriety, three decades, or three days.

Repeat after me: *It's okay. I'm okay. And I have faith that my recovery is going to be okay.*

Yet I know that affirming yourself with Unconditional Love might seem impossible after a relapse. For those of us who need and want sobriety more than anything in the world, it's devastating to let ourselves down, and to disappoint those who are counting on us to stay sober, too. That's why using your drug again after a period of sobriety, regardless of how long you've been sober, tends to trigger an emotional reflex of intense shame and regret.

I understand that self-flagellation might seem like the only logical response to the gut punch that is relapse. After all, you don't want to let yourself off the hook. Beating yourself up is meant to be a self-inflicted consequence to ensure you don't do it again.

In theory, I suppose this makes sense. In practice, however, shaming yourself is no way to facilitate positive change. So I'm still going to urge you to act as if you believe in Unconditional Love, even if you don't intellectually buy it, just yet.

Repeat after me: *It's okay. I'm okay. And I have faith that my recovery is going to be okay.*

From there, the next most helpful thing to do is to ask yourself, *how can I reach out for help?* The right kind of support, from the people who have been through what you're going through (including relapse), is going to help you stop using and start believing in yourself. In my experience, person-to-person support has a way of righting your sobriety ship even more powerfully than repeating affirmations into the mirror by yourself does. There's something about hearing another person express hope for you that tends to help you actually believe those affirmations.

My dear Addict friends, I can sense you wincing from here. Why is it that most of us would rather drink a ground-glass smoothie than tell another human being we need help? Pride and shame are the number one offenders.

I should be able to solve my problems myself! you say, bleeding from the eyes as you stagger under the crushing weight of Your Addict, so stalwartly determined to hide your relapse. You know how that sentence ends, though? *...and I'll die trying!*

So stop it. First of all, you can't do recovery by yourself. That's a fantasy cooked up by Your Addict, that disingenuous bastard, who wants you to stay alone — and addicted — in the dark. The last thing it wants is for you to call in outside reinforcement to help kick its ass.

Think of it this way: if you could stay sober without asking for help, then how come Your Addict's not hog-tied and helpless in the corner already? Sobriety means doing a hard thing, and like a lot of hard things, it's way too hard to do all on your own. You're gonna need help from other humans, and that's okay. More than okay, actually. It's ideal. That's because being honest about needing help is yet another expression of Unconditional Love for Your True Self.

Remember: Unconditional Love is the ultimate healing agent in recovery, as in life.

All that being said, I need to address what tends to be our biggest hangup, post-relapse, when it comes to asking for help from other recovering addicts. There's a reason it can feel so scary to go back to your recovery meetings and tell the truth about your relapse, even in the name of helping yourself get sober again.

Fear of judgment.

We addicts tend to have a hair-trigger sensitivity to the slightest whiff of judgment, and we react to it like it's outright condemnation. If your history is anything like mine, you've done some pretty crazy things to retaliate against the judgment of others, or to avoid coming into contact with it altogether. Either way, defensive reactions are usually a projection of the shame and judgment we're harboring about ourselves, as opposed to any real threat posed by the opinions of others.

I promise, they're not thinking about you nearly as much as you're thinking about yourself.

I do, though, want to get up on my soapbox and comment about one aspect of the fear-of-judgment-in-recovery-meetings issue that can feel extra intimidating after a relapse. That is, the obsessive focus in so many recovery fellowships — I'm looking at you, Twelve Step — on what's known as *continuous sobriety.*

Continuous sobriety is exactly what it sounds like: an uninterrupted chain of days, months, or years during which you didn't use your drug (or, depending on your definition of sobriety, any drug). Recovery meetings are typically full of people celebrating anniversaries of continuous sobriety, whether that's thirty days, six months, one year, or twelve years — and everything in between and beyond.

First off, let me say that continuous sobriety is fabulous. It's admirable. It's a huge accomplishment. It represents the triumph of escaping your prison, and not going back. And it happens to be critical to the health and welfare of so many of us recovering addicts. That's the primary reason I urge everyone I work with to aim for maintaining continuous sobriety. Including myself.

It's easier to stay sober than it is to start over, another popular recovery expression goes. And for some, it's truly a matter of life and death.

The problem I have, though, is when an obsession with continuous sobriety ends up fostering an excess of relapse-related shame and despair. You have no idea how many times I've seen a client come in sobbing because they drank a bottle of wine over the weekend after finding out some terrible news — or whatever else might have prompted their relapse.

There's no way I can face all those people with years and years of sobriety in my meetings, they'll say, miserably. *They're going to be so disappointed in me.*

Okay, right off the bat, let's remind ourselves that this is exactly what recovery meetings are for — to help addicts stop using. *The only requirement for membership is a desire to stop* [using our drug], is how my own Twelve Step fellowship begins every meeting. Please note that this is very different from, *you have to be sober a long time to be eligible to receive our support.*

But I've been there myself, so I know how dreadful it can feel to come back to meetings after a relapse, or in the midst of one.

True, there may be a couple of sanctimonious jerks who say something unhelpful, like, *better you than me!* There may also be those people who go off on an unsolicited lecture that prominently features the phrase *you just need to...* [insert their personal relapse prevention wisdom]. That kind of stuff can be annoying as hell, which is why the Mama Bear in me wants to march right into your next recovery meeting with you and personally take out anyone who so much as gives you a side eye, let alone a *tsk tsk*, when you talk about your relapse.

Then again, I also know that you're going to be accepted and encouraged at those meetings infinitely more than you would ever be chastised or patronized. So much of our fear of judgment ends up being fantasy, a projection of our own guilt and shame. And as I've said before, the number one way to diminish the shame that rouses Your Addict's appetite is to turn it over to the light of Unconditional Love. Dispel that shame by being honest with others about it.

Just don't allow your goal of continuous sobriety to backfire in the form of self-sabotaging shame, if and when you veer away from that goal. An obsession with continuous sobriety tends to make the matter of relapse far too black and white for recovering addicts.

I mean, there are relapses, and then there are *relapses.*

For example, using your drug on four separate days over the course of your first year of recovery might feel shameful and demoralizing — as in, *oh man, four relapses? I suck!* But I would urge you to step back and put it in perspective. Pre-recovery, you were probably using your drug every day, or close to it. So come on... 361 out of 365 ain't bad! In fact, it's downright awesome.

The other shame-laced sentiment I tend to hear from recovering addicts who have relapsed is, *I guess this means I'm back at square one, now.*

Woof. You're not in a hole, my dear Addict friends — not even if your relapse meant a painful landing on a new rock bottom. You've got experience under your belt in recovery now, and what you've learned about yourself along the way hasn't gone anywhere. The only question is whether you're willing to pick yourself up and keep walking this road, or if you're going to allow shame and discouragement to drive you back to using again indefinitely.

So no, you are not back at square one, not even if you're having trouble getting sober again after a relapse. Now you know the steps to take: admitting your powerlessness over your drug; accepting that you're in the midst of a process that is still very much in process; and reaching out for the help you need to get back on track. Maybe that means loading up on recovery meetings every day, or maybe it means pursuing intensive professional treatment. Or both.

The bottom line on relapse is that it only means what you decide it means. Will it be a blessing, in that it ultimately moves you to a place of deeper acceptance of your powerlessness over your drug, and a deeper commitment to giving Unconditional Love to Your True Self? Or will you use it as a reason to withdraw from the process of learning how to love, and revert to unquestioning surrender to Your Addict's rotten, restrictive regime?

Remember, whether you're sober or still using your drug, you're only on the outside of recovery if you want to be. The only requirement to walk this road is the desire to love and live as Your True Self.

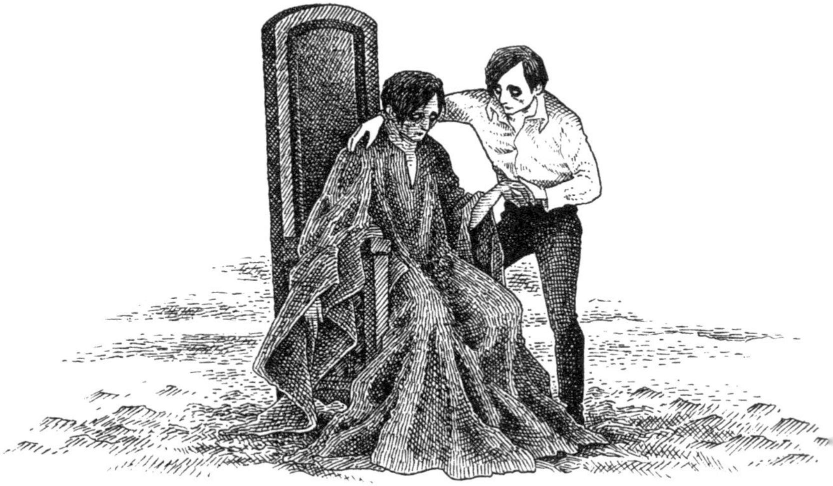

SECTION 3

GETTING WITH THE PROGRAM

CHAPTER 14

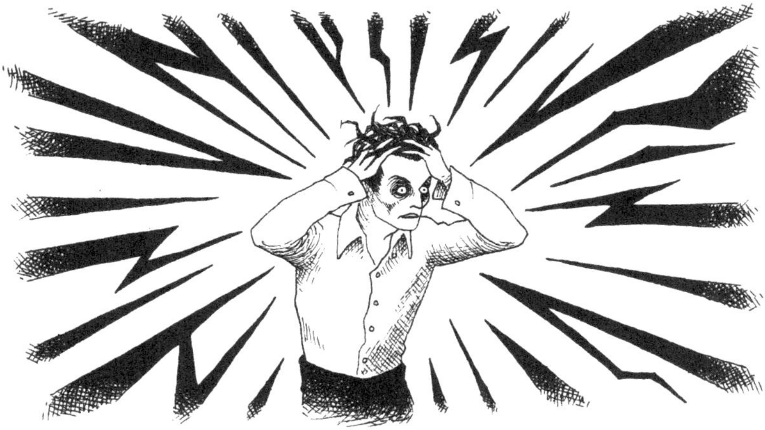

The Gift of Desperation

There's an old expression that pretty well sums up how addicts feel once we decide we need to get sober. As well as once we start getting sober. Oh, and once we actually are sober.

Restless, irritable, and discontent. (Also known as *itchy, bitchy, and twitchy.*)

This revolving door of terrible emotions feels like the oppressive weight of *blah,* alternating with your nervous system screaming *screw you!* and topped with a crushing blow of *I feel terrible but I also can't seem to do anything but sit here and keep feeling terrible.*

Whether you're aware of it or not, feeling restless, irritable, and discontent is your emotional reaction to some stone-cold reality, staring you dead in the eye. You're aware that you can't keep living in steady decline, on your knees and at the mercy of your drug. But you also can't comprehend, let alone visualize, let alone have faith in, a life without your drug.

Talk about being stuck between Your Addict and a hard place.

Face it: your comfort zone is no longer comfortable, and that makes you *restless*. The prospect of undergoing a huge life change is both utterly unknown and unequivocally unavoidable, and that makes you *irritable*. And staring gloomily into the void left behind by your drug makes you deeply *discontent*.

My dear Addict friends, are you struggling with any or all of the feelings in this toxic trio? Are they lining up like three cherries in a row after a lucky yank on a slot machine? If so, then I'm going to propose that you consider yourself lucky. Yes, really. Lucky.

I know, I know. You can't imagine where I'm going with this, because right now, you feel anything but lucky.

I'm serious, though. If you're struggling with these massively uncomfortable feelings, it means you've got a huge leg up on the addicts who are only sorta uncomfortable. Or worse, the addicts who are still sitting pretty in the sandbox of denial, just before a Sahara-worthy sandstorm starts blowing up in their face.

You, on the other hand, have made it beyond those stages of doomed, delusional ignorance. Congratulations on being officially post-reality check; you've got the restless, irritable, and discontent feelings to prove it. Now, instead of allowing those feelings to hold you hostage, you can start using them to your advantage in the way that only a deep awareness of the truth can.

Look down at your lap right now, because there's a beautifully wrapped gift sitting right under your nose. It's called *the gift of desperation.*

Yes, I understand that nobody likes to think of themselves as desperate. Desperation calls to mind the sort of pathetic soul who runs around like a chicken with its head cut off, lurching toward its next life failure in a long series of failures. *Desperate* may not seem to describe you, especially if favorable circumstances have earned you the dubious distinction of being a high-functioning addict.

Make no mistake, though. An addict's life can be functioning quite well on the surface while they're falling to pieces on the inside. Having a good job, a good family, good teeth, and no criminal record never excluded anyone from being emotionally desperate.

I say desperation is a gift because it's the most persuasive evidence you could possibly have for the fact that whatever you've been doing to help yourself isn't working, hasn't been working, and probably won't ever work. There is simply no way forward that you know of — and you know it.

Accepting the truth that you're fresh out of ideas and at the end of your road is a good thing, I promise. Only then do you stand a chance of opening your heart and mind to finding a different road.

This section is all about that different road. The road that is the best and only alternative I know of to the loneliness, the shame, and the insanity of addiction. It's the road that helps you weather the identity crisis that seems to go hand-in-hand with early recovery, along with all those restless, irritable, and discontent feelings. And it's the road that leads to a love-filled life as Your True Self.

There's a catch, though. This new road will challenge you. It will confront you with long-avoided truths that might put you on the defensive. It will provoke feelings of acute awkwardness on a regular basis. It will prompt you to hold your nose as you swallow some super-size helpings of humble pie. And it'll push you into taking gigantic leaps of faith into the great unknown.

There's an expression therapists often use that goes something along the lines of, *people are only ready to change when the pain of staying the same seems greater than the pain of change.*

My dear Addict friends, I know the feeling.

After all, I come to you as a fellow addict, through and through. I'll tell you my story here and in the chapters that follow, because even though I still feel twinges of embarrassment at certain elements of it, being honest about the true nature of My Addict is the only way I can overcome the shame that almost killed My True Self.

And honesty is still the way I access the Unconditional Love I need to live.

Let's start with all the gateway drugs My Addict originally fed on. There was alcohol, for the better part of two decades, along with cocaine and Ecstasy, in my hard-partying, post-college days. Then there were the pills: the anti-anxiety meds Klonopin and Xanax, the prescription sleep aid Ambien, and the stimulant drug Ritalin, in my twenties and into my early thirties.

My Addict loved to do those drugs. My Addict loved to drink. I was certainly addicted to them all, for the way they took away my power and brought on so much out-of-control behavior and despair. But I was able to stop using each one of them in succession, without too much fanfare. None of them brought me to the brink of emotional breakdown and psychological collapse, or hog-tied my free will and shoved my face in a stinking mess of shame and self-loathing, even close to the way marijuana did.

Seriously! *Weed.*

I know, right? After all those years of abusing alcohol and drugs, weed revealed itself to be My Addict's true drug of choice. And I lived for so long in so much pain and so much insanity, unable to stop using it, because nobody knew.

Nobody knew, so nobody could understand, so nobody could help me.

Weed is a funny drug. It's being legalized all over the place, which means it's being normalized all over the place. Dispensaries are now as ubiquitous as liquor stores in Michigan, which is just over the border from me, in Indiana. Grandmas eat weed gummies for a bit of fun and relaxation. Cancer patients use it to get their appetite back. Chronic pain sufferers smoke to find relief.

I get that there are lots of reasons weed is increasingly available these days. I get that there are people who can enjoy weed recreationally, then take it or leave it every other day of the week. There is no possible world I can conceive of in which I am one of those people, however.

There's even a conventional wisdom that suggests weed is not addictive, or that its negative effects are confined to eating too much junk food and giggling uncontrollably. Yet I have volumes of tear-stained, angst-ridden journals that speak directly to the despair and insanity of a hardcore weed addiction like mine.

When weed is in my life, it quickly takes over my life. My Addict seizes upon weed as an all-around solution to my day-to-day problems, for the way it catapults me to a fantasy land in which I am not really myself, and things and people around me appear different from the way they really are. My Addict insists that my real life will never be as awesome as that fantasy land, so it obsesses about when it can get back there again.

That obsession took the form of incessant calculations — while I was in the shower, at work, driving to the store, or playing with my kids. If I was conscious, I was probably plotting my next high.

When am I going to smoke weed again?
How much am I going to buy?
How much am I going to smoke?
Where can I go off to smoke so I can successfully hide it?
Which people can I be around stoned and get away with it?

And so on. You'd have thought weed was my lover, the way I schemed and dreamed about being alone with it, away from prying eyes. Yet I hated weed for what it was doing to me.

I hated how weed turned me into a stinky, bloated, stumbling mess of a person. I hated how weed took away my integrity in my career as an addiction and recovery therapist. I hated how weed disconnected me from my kids, even when we were in the same room together. I hated how weed stole my money, betrayed me, then had me craving and chasing it again the very next day.

God, how I hated weed — along with My Addict, for the way it demanded weed, and how it always manipulated me into going back to it. My Addict would sneer at me one minute for having a problem with weed, then overpower all my convictions to quit using it the next.

Remember how I talked about how terrible Your Addict is with problems, though? How it refuses to ask for help as it does nothing but obsess about the problem? And how all that obsessing doesn't solve the problem, it just makes the problem seem inseparable from you?

That's exactly what happened to me. At a certain point, I felt like I had only one identity: My Addict, which was growing stronger and stronger, and which I hated more and more with each successive day I used weed. That meant I spent all day, every day, unable to stop using weed, and hating myself.

I've heard it said that shame only lives in the dark — under conditions of secrecy and isolation. For me, that was literally true. I remember many afternoons spent in the darkness of my bedroom, the curtains pulled to block any intrusive light. I had a THC vape pen in one hand, and a pillow in the other to muffle my sobs. Each time I inhaled, I asked myself bitterly, *which came first, the weed or the self-loathing?*

It was hard to say which one I hated more: weed, for what it was doing to me, or My Addict, for being unable to put that vape pen down.

And when I say I couldn't put it down, I mean it. I carried that little vape pen in the back pocket of my jeans, surreptitiously taking hits until I was so stoned and disgusted with myself, I'd throw the whole thing away — in a garbage can across town, that is, so I wouldn't be tempted to dig it out of my own trash in a few hours. That might work to stop me from smoking overnight, but the following morning I'd be back to buy a new vape pen and THC cartridge, which would start the whole cycle of using and self-loathing all over again.

To switch things up a bit, I'd buy actual weed and smoke it in a glass pipe until I got so stoned and disgusted with myself, I'd flush the rest down the toilet and break the pipe for good measure. Then I'd peer into the bowl anxiously, telling myself that if there was still a bud floating around after the flush, I was allowed to fish it out and let it dry before smoking again. In the broken pipe.

So much insanity. So much shame. So much wasted time, money, and emotional energy. So why wasn't I getting help? I guess you could say My Addict was pretty cunning at finding ways to keep me alone and in the dark — helpless and hopeless.

I mean, let's not ignore the headline here: I was an addiction therapist with an active addiction. My Addict told me that it was impossible to ask for help. It told me that if I was honest with another therapist, they would report me to the licensing board. It told me that all my clients would leave me if they found out what a hypocrite I was.

But the real answer to why it took me so long to get help was that I was afraid. Afraid of the consequences of people finding out about my stupid, shameful weed addiction, yes. But I was afraid of a lot of other things, too.

I was afraid I'd never find pleasure without weed.

I was afraid I'd never find a way to relax without weed.

I was afraid I wouldn't be as creative, or fun, or cool without weed.

I was afraid to face the day-to-day stresses of life without weed.

I was afraid to feel sadness, or loneliness, or anger without weed.

I was afraid I'd have nothing to celebrate with, without weed.

Emotionally, I was afraid I'd be left with nothing without weed.

And that's the bottom line of what Your Addict does to you, too. It isolates you and leaves you full of fear, so you cling even more fiercely to the drug that dragged you down to those depths. Being alone and afraid is one of the most painful feelings in the world, which is why you keep running back to your drug: to make those feelings go away.

I've already told you that love is the solution to all the fear, shame, and isolation Your Addict has beaten Your True Self to a pulp with. But I'm sorry to say that love didn't come running out of nowhere to hose me down with hearts and rainbows, like firefighters drowning out a five-alarm blaze. I think it's safe to say that it won't for you, either.

Don't get me wrong. Love is going to be there when you need it. But the step you have to take before you can get it is admitting that you need it. The gift of desperation means more than just being ready for change. It means that your heart and mind are open to being guided by something outside of yourself — something you haven't been able to give yourself just yet.

CHAPTER 15

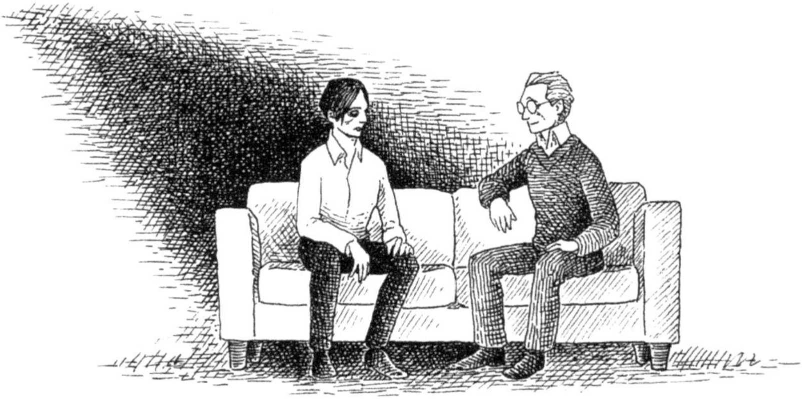

Get Yourself an Honesty Coach

My dear Addict friends, I swear, I'm not going to sit here and tell you that you absolutely must join A.A., or Narcotics Anonymous, or any other type of Twelve Step program. I'm not even going to tell you that you have to get a therapist. And I am a therapist! But I've never been the kind of therapist who gives out ultimatums. We addicts are a rebellious lot by nature, and I respect that.

But if you want to stay sober and find the peace, freedom, and happiness of living as Your True Self, I am going to give you one piece of golden advice.

Get yourself an honesty coach.

Go ahead and search it up. You won't find much. In fact, I might have made up that term when I worked with my own honesty coach. I even told him that's what I considered him to be. And if I remember correctly, he agreed immediately that an honesty coach was exactly what I needed.

But I'm getting ahead of myself. Let me start from the beginning.

I found my honesty coach by doing a search for "addiction counselor near me." Before my first appointment, he asked me to email him a description of the problem that made me seek him out. This is what I wrote:

I'm feeling overwhelmed. I need to prioritize. I need to weed out toxic people from my life.

It's not that those were lies, exactly. But it certainly wasn't the truth. Oh, wait. There was one true word in it: *weed*. See, my real problem — the problem I didn't write down at the time — was that I needed to get sober from weed.

Now let's get back to my honesty coach. He happened to be a therapist, like me. But he was also a therapist who had at least a dozen years of sobriety on me. A therapist whose placid demeanor was the epitome of laid-back serenity. A therapist I could barely stand to be in the same room with, that first year I was meeting with him.

I used to do everything I could to avoid getting honest with the guy. I'd spend our sessions talking about my childhood. Or the guy I was always breaking up and getting back together with. Or my writing projects. Anything but my weed addiction.

I'd also try to avoid him by cancelling our sessions at the last minute. Or I'd tiptoe around the issues I didn't want to talk about, as though they were land mines about to detonate if I made one wrong move. And you're gonna love this one: I lied to him. Imagine! Me, a therapist, lying to my therapist. Worse — lying to my honesty coach.

See? I told you I needed an honesty coach.

The thing was, I did eventually admit to him how badly I needed to stop smoking weed. My honesty coach agreed wholeheartedly that I needed to stop smoking weed, too. There was just one problem: I didn't stop smoking weed. And I lied to my honesty coach by telling him I wasn't using it.

Are you scratching your head at that? Or are you just as much of an addict as I am? Which is to say, do you completely understand why I was lying to my honesty coach?

That's right. I didn't want to be sober.

As crazy and counterproductive as it sounds, lying to my honesty coach enabled me to keep using my drug. But that wasn't the only reason I was lying. After all, I could have just told him, flat out, *I want to keep smoking weed even though I know I shouldn't be smoking weed.* That wouldn't have been a lie at all!

My friends, there are many ways to be an addict. But whether your addiction is to alcohol, or some other drug, or gambling, or porn, or sugar, or video games, there is one core addiction we all have in common.

Control.

We addicts needed to control our mood — whether that was boredom, loneliness, anger, anxiety, or even excitement — with our drug. Having that control allowed us to escape our feelings, our thoughts, our problems, and ultimately, ourselves.

But that's not the only thing we tried to control. We twisted ourselves up in knots trying to control plenty of other people, places, and things, under the sadly misguided notion that we could. I know I used to try to control what other people thought. How they felt. And especially, what they thought and how they felt about me.

That brings me back to the answer of why I lied to my honesty coach. I was terrified of him seeing me at my most out of control. So I did what addicts do when they're afraid, and they desperately want to control their fear.

They hide.

Initially, I'd hidden from my own truth that I was powerless over weed, and how much damage it was doing to my life. Then I started hiding from my honesty coach — at first by lying and withholding, and later by literally hiding. I stopped seeing him for the better part of six months, with no explanation. Wait, scratch that. I did explain, but the explanation I gave him was a lie. Fancy that!

I probably don't need to tell you that my life did not get better, those six months I went into hiding. And it probably won't surprise you that I did not stop smoking weed during those six months, either. Not even after I told myself I

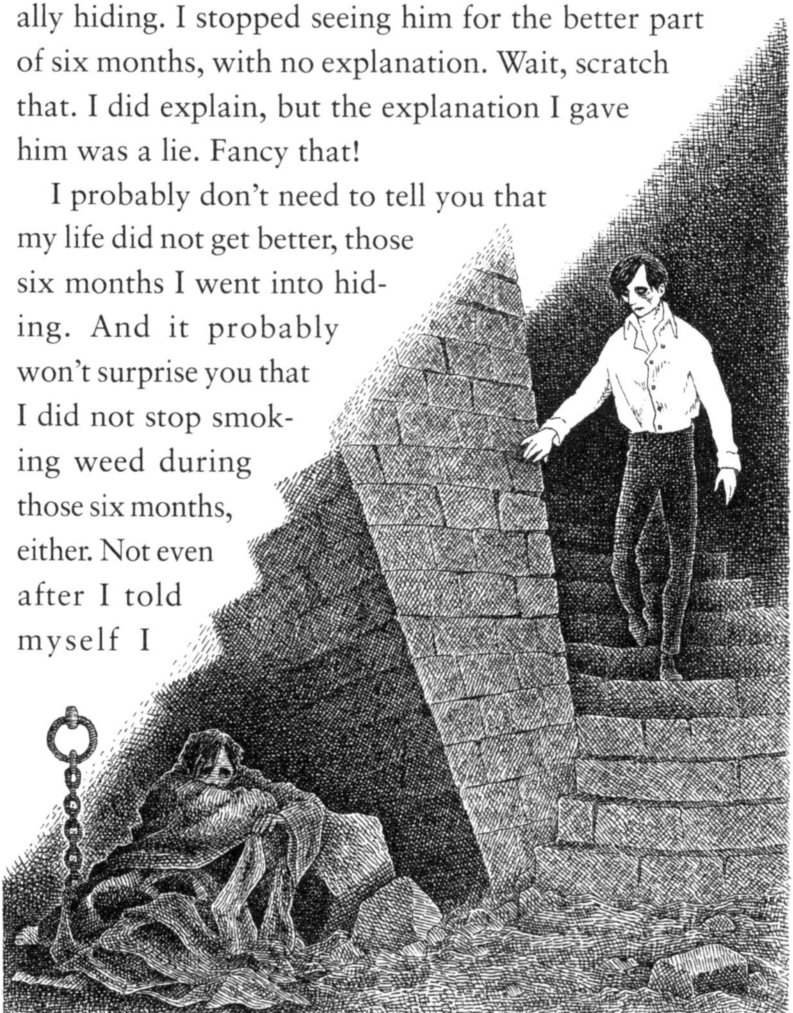

had to. Not even after I swore I could do it on my own, and that I had it all under control.

I don't remember the rock-bottom event that prompted me to reach out to my honesty coach again. I just remember sobbing in my car, in a CVS parking lot, before pulling out my phone in an act of sheer desperation.

Can we meet again? I texted him.

Sure, he replied. Just like that! As if I were a normal, human person, instead of a shitty, lying addict stuck to the bottom of his shoe.

Before we met again, I wrote him a letter. It was the letter where I let go of all the control I wanted over how my honesty coach saw me, the control I never really had in the first place. It was the letter where I started being honest.

> *I need your help. And by 'help,' I mean, a lot of help. I am way past the point of frustration. Way past the point of pride, hangups, or shame about this insane problem. My addiction. I have been totally unable to quit. And I want this letter to signal my willingness, right now. I am committing myself to sobriety, which means I am committing myself to our work together. I need you to tell me exactly what to do to be successful. I need to avail myself of all your knowledge. Whatever you got, I will listen and apply it in the fierce hope that it*

can work for me, too. I also need you to remind me to have faith in sobriety, because you are someone I trust. Which is rare.

After I watched my wafer-thin ego go up in smoke, I started seeing my honesty coach again. Only this time, I committed to being completely honest with him.

The first and most important thing I had to be honest about was that I needed help. I mean, obviously. But I had to say it to him, which was humiliating. At least, it was for the first few minutes, before utter relief kicked in.

Next up on the truth-telling agenda was admitting to my honesty coach that I'd been lying about using for most of the time I'd known him. He told me that wasn't a shameful thing. It was just a symptom of My Addict controlling me and doing everything it could to protect itself, as long as I was feeding it.

Then I had to tell my honesty coach the truth that I was just as afraid of getting sober as I was desperate to get sober. Not that I really had to say it. My fears spoke for themselves whenever I let myself cry in front of him, which got to be every single time I saw him. Clearly, my feelings were another important part of my truth I had to deal with.

I don't want to give the impression that my honesty coach was just a passive receptacle for my honesty, though. One of the most helpful things he did was to shine a terrifyingly bright flashlight onto any dark, shadowy corners of truth that I might still be trying to conceal. He'd look me right in the eye at the beginning of each session and ask me, point blank, *have you been using, Emily?*

After I gave him my answer, he'd tack on a double whammy of a truth challenge. *Are you telling me the truth about that?*

But wait, there's more! After we'd finished a session, I couldn't beat my retreat before having to answer his hideous parting question. *Is there anything you haven't told me the truth about today?*

Indeed, my honesty coach had a way of shaking the truth out of me like loose change from an old purse. But it wasn't just the truth that came out. The dead weight of shame that surrounded so much of my truth came loose, too, in waves of merciful relief.

I'm happy to say that six weeks after I sent my honesty coach that first honest letter, I finally stopped smoking weed — for what I fervently believe is for good. One day at a time, of course, as he would be the first to remind me.

It's not that my honesty coach did the work of getting sober for me. No one can do that for you, either. But he knew the truth about how much I needed to be sober. How much I wanted to be sober. And he cared enough to want me to be sober, too. That's why he challenged me to keep telling the truth, and to keep staying true to my truth.

It's been a few years, and I don't see my honesty coach anymore. I'd like to think that's because I graduated from ıching with an advanced degree in honesty, but that wouldn't be the truth at all. I just went from having one honesty coach to having multiple coaches — most of whom have no idea they're coaching me at all.

What I mean is that I'm committed to bringing my honesty to all my relationships these days.

Let me be clear, though. That doesn't mean it's gotten easier to tell the truth, especially where it counts. Dropping honesty bombshells still makes me want to run and hide in the corner with my fingers in my ears and my eyes squeezed shut, like I'm anticipating a nuclear explosion in response.

The last thing I want is for the people I love to look at me with confusion, or annoyance, or anxiety. I want so much to control what they see by presenting the prettiest and least challenging version of myself. For their comfort and convenience, of course.

Wait, that's a lie. Nine times out of ten, withholding the truth is really for my own comfort and convenience. Sure, I might tell myself that what I'm about to tell them won't be okay with them. But by and large, the only person my truth isn't okay with is me. I still have to remind myself that my feelings of shame don't mean that my truth is unacceptable. It just makes my truth a thing I'm gonna need some help with.

As painful as it is, I believe that telling your truth to another person is the only way you can start to recognize the parts of your life that don't make sense. The parts that aren't working. The parts you need to heal. The parts you need to start taking care of.

Telling the truth is about surrendering that carefully constructed image of who you think you are, and who you think you should be. It's about deconstructing the façade you've spent a lifetime cultivating. But let me ask you, haven't you lied, cheated, and twisted yourself up in knots trying to protect that image, thinking all the while that you were protecting yourself?

Unfortunately, protecting that image is what keeps the truth of you hidden and hurting, and completely unable to trust yourself. Your own decisions. Your own thoughts. Your own feelings. Even your own pain.

But I'm here to tell you that all that shit is real. All that shit is true. And not telling the truth doesn't make that truth go away. Quite the opposite. An untold truth is a truth that haunts you, in all sorts of crazy ways. Lying and pretending and protecting your image — you know, the one in which you're a fully functioning person who's *doing just fine on my own, thanks!* — only amounts to you betraying yourself.

Your True Self.

Recovery, on the other hand, is about surrendering the weapon that's killing you: your shame about the truth of yourself. For most addicts, recovery feels like the first chance we've had at learning to accept and be true to ourselves — at least, since we were brand new to the world. Back before we stopped trusting ourselves, and became capable of hiding.

While you're learning to trust your own truth again, you're going to need the sense of safety that comes from unconditional acceptance, as well as the sense of being cared for that comes from trust and consistency. Recovering addicts who participate in a Twelve Step fellowship often find that caring honesty coach by working with what's known as a *sponsor*. A sponsor functions as their confidante and mentor in guiding them through the Twelve Steps of recovery.

Others of us don't want a sponsor (or don't do Twelve Step programs at all), which is fine, too. Hire that caring honesty coach if you can, like I did. Ideally, your coach would be a fellow recovering addict who's farther along the road of their own truth-telling journey, but it's not a dealbreaker if they're not. A counselor you trust and can meet with regularly, and who keeps you honest and accountable, is far, far better than no honesty coach at all.

Just please, don't leave yourself totally unsupervised in your very first days, weeks, and months of recovery. I mean, would you really expect a newborn baby to take care of itself? Wouldn't it need guidance, encouragement, and someone it could trust to help it navigate its brand new life, and overcome its fears?

You do, too.

CHAPTER 16

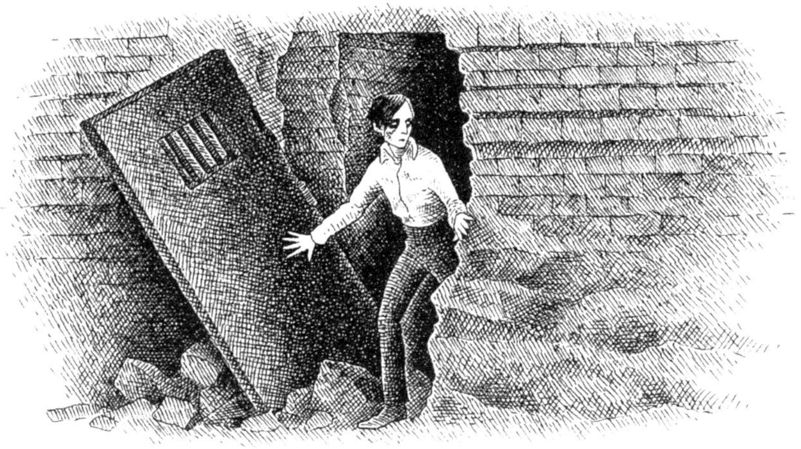

The Security of Structure

There's no big magical mystery in what addiction therapy is all about. In fact, I can sum it up in a single sentence: *helping people become liberated from their own prisons of fear.*

Or if that's too complicated, I can do it in one word: *freedom.*

The thing about freedom, though, is that it's not as easy to enjoy as most people believe. Personally, I think freedom is the number one scariest thing about life in general. I mean, I've seen a lot of people flunk out of freedom.

I used to work as a group therapist for guys who had just gotten out of jail or prison, leading a program called Moral Reconation Therapy. MRT started out in correctional facilities back in the 1980s, and it was designed to help criminal offenders make good decisions and get their lives together. The program emphasizes staying sober, setting goals, and taking total responsibility for your life.

The MRT workbook features an ominous picture of a jail cell on the cover, and the title doesn't beat around the bush, either: *How to Escape Your Prison.*

As a therapist, I was big into MRT because it was fun, but also hardcore. It was like *Fight Club* for addicts, if you swapped the beatdowns for some highly moral decision making. And if you had me instead of Tyler Durden cheering you on.

But MRT was just as liberating and just as character-building — as long as the guys put in the honest work of change. The motto of the program was, *the more you play by the rules, the more freedom you will have.* When I'd write that across the top of the white board in all caps, it got some confused looks from new guys. But it wasn't long before they understood what it meant.

For them, following the rules literally meant freedom.

When it came to rules, MRT had a few non-negotiables. Everyone in the group had to live by those rules if they wanted to finish MRT, which they were required to, or risk violating their parole and getting locked up again. One of the guys, Wayne, made us a poster with all the rules written in big magic marker.

#5: What happens in MRT, stays in MRT.
#4: No arguing with anyone.
#3: Respect yourself, others, and your leader.
#2: No drugs or alcohol.
#1: Honesty.

Are you taking notes? Because those are good rules for any recovering addict, criminal record or not.

There was no question that the first thing you were required to do in MRT was the hardest: Testimony. And that's exactly what it was. The new guy had to stand at the front of the room in front of everyone, which was terrifying in itself. Then, without a script or notes to prompt him, he had to be as honest as he could in explaining how he ended up in MRT. He'd conclude his Testimony by telling everyone that he was committed to changing his life.

Like everything else in MRT, change was not optional.

Your typical new guy had no idea what he was doing in his Testimony, and by that I mean he had no idea how to be honest, let alone how to take responsibility for his actions, let alone how to commit to the process of positive personal change. And everyone knew it. After he finished his Testimony, he'd have to leave the room while the other guys took a vote about whether he'd passed the step. Two out of three times, they'd tell him to come back next week and try it again.

He was lying about everything, blaming all his shit on other people, the MRT veterans would say. *He's not ready to change yet.*

It could take a new guy a full month to get real enough to convince the group that he should keep going in MRT. But as humbling as the Testimony was, everyone knew that the purpose of the program wasn't to humiliate them, or to change them from being "bad guys" into "good guys."

The purpose of MRT was to teach them how to be honest. How to take responsibility for their problems, so they could actually work on them. And how to set and pursue goals so they could make their lives better. Happier. Freer.

For your typical addict ex-con, though, freedom wasn't a fun little choose-your-own-adventure kind of deal. It was a crashing boulder of reality that had just landed squarely on his shoulders. After being told for years where to go and what to do — or, as the guys liked to put it, *when to shit, shower, and shave* — he'd been thrust into an indifferent world to fend for himself.

As the MRT group leader, I tried my best to support them, but not everyone made it. Our graduation rate was pretty good, but it was what happened after they left the program that mattered.

I still get choked up when I think about a guy I'll call William, a dreadlocked 25-year-old who'd come to group every week in a three-piece suit to show how serious he was about self-improvement. A few months after we threw William a pizza party for his MRT graduation, I saw an article in the local news about him. He'd been shot and killed while allegedly trying to break into an apartment.

The prospect of doing life honestly, without breaking the law, seemed next to impossible for a lot of guys. I remember another one I'll call Eddie, who'd come to group after a twelve-hour factory shift with his head hanging down like a hound dog, dark circles under his eyes. He was always trying to find a place to live, or trying to find rides to work. But mostly, he was trying to stay away from selling and using cocaine.

Maaaaaaaaan, I can still picture Eddie saying, as he'd flop down into one of the chairs in the group circle. *Imma bout to giiiiiive up. This shit is no joke.*

By which he meant, *responsibility is no joke.* Neither was stealing, hustling, hurting himself, abandoning his kids, or going to prison, he'd be the first to tell you. But at least the unwritten rules of the street were a defined way to live. Without those, he felt as vulnerable as a baby bunny.

Is this starting to sound familiar to any of you out there in early sobriety? The thing about Your Addict was that it imprisoned you in one hell of a daily routine, and you clung to it like flypaper. You carried out its orders like a good little soldier, even as you cursed your drug for making you stuck and miserable.

That's why it always strikes me as ironic to hear addicts hating on recovery programs that emphasize the importance of living by your own personal "higher power." Is that idea really more offensive or outlandish than the way your drink, your drug, or some other addictive higher power ruled your life, dictating when you were allowed to shit, shower, and shave?

The fact is, it's human nature to seek security in structure, no matter how dysfunctional that structure is, or how counterproductive its rules are. On a subconscious level, it's a relief to be told what to do by our friends and family, or by our employers, or by larger-than-life institutions, or by societal and cultural expectations. The alternative — freedom — is a lot of responsibility. If we fail, we have no one to blame but ourselves.

Just like people on parole, recovering addicts in early sobriety tend to feel overwhelmed and unprepared when the day-to-day structure of pursuing our drug is no longer there. To shield ourselves from the responsibility of freedom, we seek refuge in every defense mechanism in the psychological playbook. We act helpless. We isolate ourselves. We play the victim. We hide behind the most limiting interpretation of the disease model of addiction. Sometimes after we get sober, our instinct is to retreat from life and sit slumped with our head in our hands, like Eddie. We can't understand why everything still feels so difficult to manage.

What you've got to understand, my dear Addict friends, is that getting sober from your drug marks your release from your own kind of prison, after years of incarceration. That leaves you unmoored and adrift, which translates to feeling lonely, confused, and overwhelmed.

What you need is the safety and structure of a *recovery program.*

Look, I don't like the word "program" any more than you don't. It's right up there with people talking about the "work" of recovery, when it comes to no-fun words that make me groan. The idea of *getting with the program* — any program — might send chills down your spine. But I hope you'll come to embrace it.

The idea is for your recovery program to become truly your own, so it starts to feel less and less like a straitjacket Nurse Ratchet is trying to wrangle you into, and more and more like a comfy pair of sweatpants you make a beeline to seek refuge in.

The ultimate structure when it comes to recovery programs, of course, is inpatient treatment, otherwise known as *rehab*. Rehab means leaving your home for thirty, sixty, or ninety days, and staying at a treatment facility where you have no access to your drug. Instead, nearly every minute of every day is structured for you. There's a mandatory wake-up time. Mandatory meals. Mandatory group therapy. Mandatory individual therapy. Mandatory art therapy, mandatory yoga, mandatory movie night, mandatory Twelve Step meetings, and a host of other mandatory activities to ensure you don't have a minute left open to succumb to Your Addict's mandates.

The next most structured kind of recovery program is what's known as Intensive Outpatient (IOP) treatment. The specifics of IOP programs vary, but they generally consist of an eight to twelve-week intensive phase, during which you show up at a treatment facility three days a week, for three or four hours a day. Your time there is mostly spent in group therapy, but you'll likely have some individual therapy as well. Some IOP programs include mandatory drug testing, too. Once the intensive phase is over, most IOPs offer an aftercare program that consists of weekly group therapy sessions, and maybe a weekly individual session, for anywhere from six months to a year.

Whether inpatient or outpatient, these treatment programs — which function like recovery boot camps — can be incredibly helpful. They're life-saving for addicts who would otherwise find it impossible to get a sober recovery off the ground. If that describes you, and you have the resources and the opportunity to pursue those programs, that's terrific. By all means, get with the program!

No matter how beneficial those structured treatment programs are, though, they all have one thing in common: an inevitable end. Unfortunately, many of the recovering addicts who leave take with them a false sense of security that they've already learned everything they need to know about staying sober. They might consider their recovery program to be completed. Worse, sometimes they leave under the delusion that they're healed of addiction, now that they've graduated.

I'll be just fine on my own! they insist. Famous last words.

One to three months of inpatient rehab, or twelve weeks of IOP, does not in and of itself make for a successful recovery program. It's a fabulous start, don't get me wrong. But completing rehab or IOP doesn't excuse anyone from the necessity of building their own recovery program, once treatment is over and regular life resumes.

Ask a hundred different recovering addicts what their day-to-day recovery program consists of, and you'll get a hundred different answers. Some include regular exercise.

Professional therapy. A creative hobby. Nightly journaling. Practicing the Twelve Steps. Morning meditation. Silent retreats. Volunteer service. Or that big, catch-all category, *staying busy*.

I don't mean to suggest that your recovery program has to include a hundred new healthy habits you've got to pursue breathlessly every day. Remember what I said about recovery being a process? Healthier habits will come with time, as you recognize their value to Your True Self, and you develop the authentic desire to create space for them in your daily life.

That's as opposed to imposing a bunch of ambitious new behaviors upon yourself right away, like the world's most high-stakes to-do list, then descending into a shame spiral when you fall short — which could send you right back into the welcoming arms of Your Addict.

As I look back on my days leading that MRT recovery program, it occurs to me that the most valuable element of its structure wasn't the obvious stuff. It wasn't the MRT workbook, which was chock-full of great information and assignments. It wasn't the MRT steps the guys had to progressively complete in order to graduate. It wasn't even the list of MRT rules they had to live by.

The most valuable part of the MRT structure was that those guys had to come together every week to collaborate and contribute to their common goal: *freedom*.

Meeting regularly and sharing honestly in a place

where they felt understood was what helped them ease their post-release feelings of anxiety, confusion, and loneliness. And encouraging and supporting one another was what helped them start believing in the good inside them, despite their troubled pasts. Cultivating that faith in themselves would have been inconceivable on their own, or within their dysfunctional families of origin.

Never in a million years would I have been able to pitch it to those guys without them rolling their eyes and snorting, but what they were really learning to do in that group was to *love* — both each other and themselves — in a mutually reinforcing process.

For better or worse, freedom is what you get when you let go of your drug. But in order to actually enjoy your freedom, and use it to make the most of the life ahead of you, you'll have to let go of a lot of other things, too.

Things like fear. Shame. Anger. Helplessness. Self-pity. Resistance.

These make up the basic structure of most addicts' emotional lives, even after we get sober. They're the kind of feelings that threaten to sink us into hopelessness and powerlessness again. Worse, they're the kind of feelings that hide Your True Self from yourself and those around you. That's because they prevent you from giving and receiving the gift of Unconditional Love.

The best kind of recovery program is the kind that helps you start to let go of those feelings, along with the thinking patterns and behaviors that trigger them. And not just by hammering into you, *you've got to let go of them!* Because that's kind of like saying, *just don't use your drug!*

The best kind of recovery program is the kind that's structured around the alternative to fear, shame, anger, helplessness, self-pity, and resistance.

Love.

Generally speaking, a recovery program is a dynamic and personal thing, a structure of loving and supportive people, attitudes, and actions you'll cultivate over an undefined period of time. What your recovery program will ultimately consist of will depend on the unique needs and desires that emerge from your progressive discovery of Your True Self.

But you can't discover Your True Self without the essential ingredient of honesty. You can't be honest without the essential ingredient of trust. And you can't have trust without a common bond — whether that's a bond of understanding, of purpose, of caring, or of consistency. Ideally, trust is built with all of those present.

My dear Addict friends, if there was any alternative to a recovery program that puts you in regular contact with the people who are guaranteed to understand you, who have the same purpose as you, who care about you, and who will reliably be there for you, then I would be the first to present it.

As it stands, though, I propose that your recovery program starts with one simple structure: a regular opportunity to connect to your own, soon-to-be, dear Addict friends.

CHAPTER 17

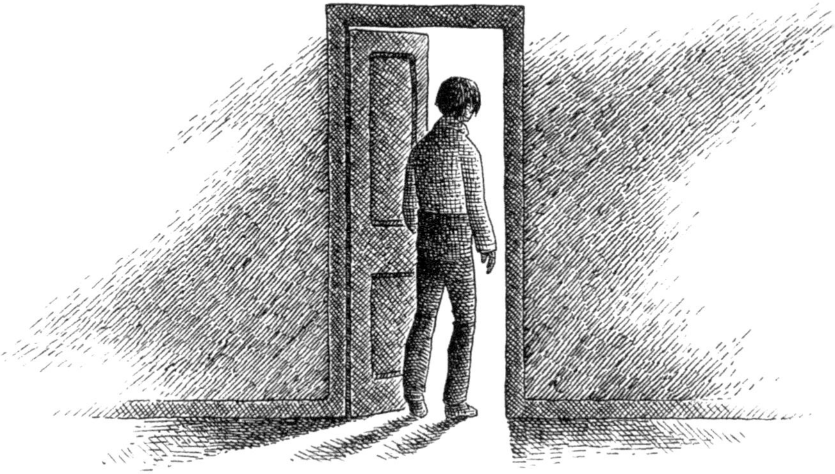

Meetings: Misery, Medicine, Magic

Let me tell you a little story about your drug, and the way your relationship with it evolved over time. Maybe "devolved" is a better word, actually.

First, your drug was *magic*. It made you feel like there were big, beautiful rainbows, hearts, and shooting stars firing off inside you. It made you tremble with excitement, and shiver with pleasure. It infused you with great big gulps of exhilaration.

Later, your drug was *medicine*. It helped you function in a way you couldn't seem to without it. Maybe it relaxed you, eased your pain, gave you courage, opened your mind, or provided much-needed stimulation and distraction from the burden of being you.

Ultimately, your drug meant *misery*. Your endless obsession with it. The steadily mounting consequences. The way it robbed you of your mental and/or physical health, your dignity, your resources, and a host of other precious things you once held dear. How it brought you to the brink of total life collapse, or at the very least, intolerable emotional desperation.

Your drug went from being magic, to medicine, to misery. Sound about right?

Well, look. I'm sorry about how that all turned out. But hey, at least now you have first-hand knowledge of how your relationship with one single thing can change so drastically over time. Keep that in mind, because your relationship with an essential element of your recovery program-to-be will likely change just as drastically, as time goes by.

Instead of a relationship that devolves and threatens

to destroy you, though, my hope is that this one evolves, and does much to enhance your Unconditional Love for Your True Self.

My dear Addict friends, it's time to talk about your relationship with *recovery meetings*. Because I'm not about to keep blathering on about how essential they are, while pretending I'm oblivious that the majority of you are wincing at the prospect of enduring such misery.

What I am going to propose, though, is the possibility that your relationship with recovery meetings could change in much the same way that the one with your drug did, except in reverse. From misery, to medicine, to magic. Imagine!

I can't tell you how many of my fellow recovering addicts tell the same story of how they started going (or not going) to meetings. How they dreaded walking into their first one so much, they sat paralyzed with anxiety in the parking lot while the meeting time came and went. For some, that had to happen more than a dozen times before they finally worked up the courage to go inside.

Maybe there's a particular aspect of recovery meetings that strikes fear and loathing into your heart. Like the act of walking into a room for the first time, in a place where you don't know anyone, and feeling everyone's eyes on you as your face burns with palpable discomfort. *Will someone I know see me here?* you wonder, terrified of being outed as an addict to the general community.

Or maybe it's the fact that you have absolutely no idea what you would say if you were required to speak during the meeting.

Maybe it's your distaste for the idea that some religious "higher power" will be pushed on you by a bunch of self-righteous nut jobs.

Or maybe it's your reluctance to associate yourself with *those people*, whom you assume will look like they came straight out of Central Casting. Perhaps you'll have to sit next to Smelly Man Who Looks Like He Lives Under a Bridge, or try to avoid the gaze of Unkempt Lady Who Mumbles to Herself in the Corner.

Maybe it's your uneasiness with the way the members introduce themselves as "addicts" or "alcoholics" — will you be expected to do the same? *Hey, maybe I'm not really an addict at all!* you get to thinking, before driving far, far away from that parking lot, perhaps even stopping to pick up your drug on the way home. (Y'know, just to prove to yourself that you're not one of them.)

Aside from fears about getting sober, it's generally the fear of identifying with other addicts that keeps people away from recovery meetings. Oh sure, you might say it's got nothing at all to do with fear or disdain. *It's a matter of principle!* you insist.

I'm not religious, and no one's going to tell me what to believe in!

My entire livelihood, and the well-being of my children,

and maybe my children's children, depends on no one ever finding out that I'm an addict!

The thing is, though, is that your conscious mind has a crafty way of throwing out any excuse it can to avoid rousing the most vulnerable, shadowy parts of yourself. Make no mistake: your list of 101 Reasons Not to Go to Recovery Meetings is typically rooted in just one reason.

Shame.

You reject being in the company of other addicts because you reject the idea that you yourself are an addict, because you reject yourself for being an addict.

Recovery meetings are scary because they threaten to trigger your most painful core belief about yourself: that *you are not okay*. Not just because you're an addict, although that doesn't do much to help your self-image. No, shame points to *you* — meaning, all of you — as the problem. Because that's what shame does. It specializes in throwing the baby out with the bathwater.

See, shame can't be compartmentalized to just one area of your life. Sure, it might have its origins in a single cause, such as childhood trauma, or sexual abuse, or addiction. But shame doesn't stop there. It seeps deep into your subconscious, darkening your entire conception of who you are.

The most insidious thing about shame is that it acts as a self-fulfilling prophecy. Your shame-based beliefs about yourself manifest as painful feelings and self-sabotaging behaviors, which sets the shame machine in motion all the more.

Is it any wonder, then, that so many would-be recovering addicts stay far away from recovery meetings, regarding them as certain misery? They intuitively sense that identifying with those people — *those addicts* — would thrust their shame into the forefront of their consciousness, causing acute emotional pain.

Of course, the problem with avoiding the most vulnerable, shadowy parts of yourself is that they'll haunt and sabotage you all the more, left to fester in the dark. I've said it before: shame is what Your Addict exploits in order to get itself fed with your drug. Shame is dangerous as hell, for the way it makes you unacceptable to yourself. It demands you do whatever it takes to hide you from yourself, as well as from other people.

Enabling shame's avoidant, self-rejecting demands will only keep you sick.

Diminishing your shame may seem like a tall order, but it is possible, with the right support. The fact that recovery meetings are that venue for shame-busting support is the number one reason I suggest that you make meetings a big part of your recovery program.

Because the thing about shame is that it's really just a big old gremlin that can only exist in the darkness of your silence and avoidance. Shame shrinks when it's thrust into the light of honesty — exponentially so, when it's met with acceptance rather than judgment. Recovery meetings are the ultimate opportunity to experience that honesty and acceptance, because they're a safe space where people share a common problem (addiction) and a common goal (recovery). Everything in between is just details.

I've seen it over and over, folks. The super-scandalous secrets you're sure will shock and sicken others will instead be met with a collective *shrug.* The fact is, your fellow recovering addicts have either heard it all before, or they've done the same scandalous things themselves.

See, every time you walk into a meeting room and stop comparing yourself to all the other addicts long enough to identify with them, you're diminishing your shame. Every time you tell your story of addiction and discover an accepting audience reflected back to you, you're diminishing your shame. Every time you find hope, or humor, or a feel-good bond of understanding in your interactions with other recovering addicts, you're diminishing your shame.

And as long as you keep attending meetings regularly, I have faith that Your Addict will begin to feel a little less powerful, a little less credible, and a little bit more like something that exists within you, as opposed to who you are. But the only way to gain that kind of clarity is to let others help you shed that suffocating cloak of shame.

For those of you who are still reluctant to attend recovery meetings, I urge you to keep an open mind to their medicinal properties, even if the initial doses feel downright miserable. Like a lot of other curative activities, like starting to exercise or eat healthfully, meetings will likely make you feel worse before they start helping you feel better.

But recovery meetings don't just help diminish the mercenary force of shame. They also help foster the most positive and protective power there is. A power you will take into yourself, carry with you, and use as a force for good in your own life, far beyond the confines of recovery meeting rooms. I'm talking about the power that feels like magic. The power that is the real prize of recovery.

Unconditional Love.

I'll tell you my own story of meeting magic, with the caveat that Unconditional Love doesn't happen for anyone in the same way. And that's part of its magic: how deeply personal it feels.

My only hope is that my story gives you hope.

CHAPTER 18

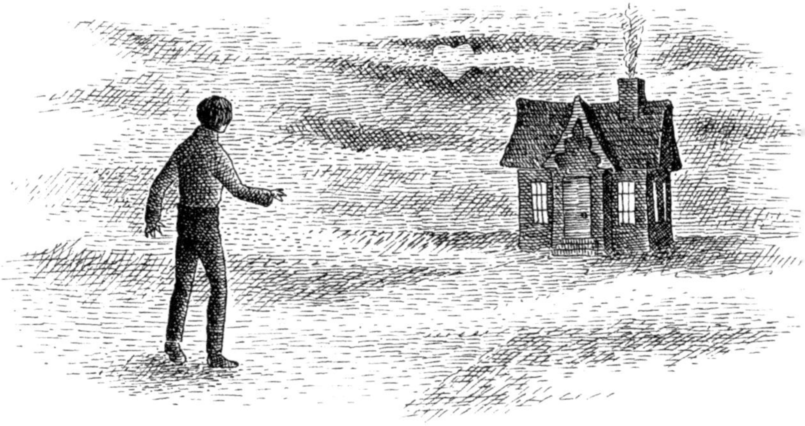

Finding Your Home

I was twenty-four the first time I fell in love. And if you've ever fallen in love, it won't surprise you that I remember everything about that momentous day. I'll clarify, though.

It wasn't love at first sight — it was love at first listen.

It was a Sunday morning, and I'd come in to work the brunch shift, hungover as usual.

Back then, I was working as a line cook at a little restaurant in the West Village of Manhattan. This was after I'd graduated from college, and walked out on two decent office jobs in the space of a year. I started working as a cook only partly because I had dreams of becoming a top chef. What I enjoyed most about it was cultivating the image of a knife-wielding, hard-partying rebel who was too edgy for some nine-to-five corporate job.

On that fateful morning, I was busy setting up my station when one of the waiters hooked up his iPod to the sound system. "Maybe it's just me," he announced to no one in particular. "But there's something about Steely Dan that just screams *brunch*."

That's when I first heard it: "Deacon Blues." It was the song I would come to know and love so deeply, over many years and many thousands of plays. The song that expressed alcoholic hopelessness as sweet romantic sorrow. With one song, Steely Dan seized me by the shoulders that hot, hungover Sunday morning, and plunged Cupid's arrow into the deepest reaches of my pop music-loving heart.

Friends of mine, who took pride in being on the cutting edge of the New York music scene, relentlessly ridiculed my love affair with Steely Dan. They lumped them in with the lame '70s crap our parents used to listen to. *Easy listening,* or what would later become known as *yacht rock*.

But there was nothing anyone could say that would dissuade me from believing that Steely Dan's music was anything but pure genius. They didn't just write songs, they told stories. Stories I could see, hear, and feel myself in. They created a whole world I could inhabit, just by listening.

Set against the backdrop of New York or L.A., your typical Steely Dan song summoned the shady side of humanity. But their songs also painted portraits of complicated people with many dimensions, both hero and antihero, over the course of a single verse. There were drug dealers. Con men. Disgraced women. Shameless lotharios. Even neighborhood pornographers.

It might go without saying that drugs and booze played a role in the music of Steely Dan, too. Scotch whiskey. Cuervo Gold. Rum and Coke. Cherry wine. Even Kirschwasser, which I had to do first-hand research to discover was a horrible-tasting cherry liqueur.

In retrospect, I can see that Steely Dan wrote their fair share of cautionary tales into their songs about flagrant drinking and drugging. But the way I was hearing it, drugs and alcohol were either a necessary anesthesia, or a sweet ambrosia, to buffer the indignities of modern life. I mean, I would — because that was me back then, an aimless dilettante set loose on lower Manhattan. I was a girl who guzzled booze and gobbled pills like they were soda pop and penny candy, all the while believing she was tragically cool for being so terminally disaffected.

I was the kind of girl who was blissfully unaware that it wasn't exactly normal to walk barefoot down Sixth Avenue at 3am after losing both her wallet and her shoes in an alcoholic blackout. Or to get in a car with a band of merry strangers and go zipping off to some faraway borough, because she just couldn't bear for the party to end when the clubs closed down at dawn.

Not long after I discovered Steely Dan, though, I burned out on New York City. The good times were losing their luster, and the crashes that followed my party girl antics were starting to pile up on me. Running low on both cash and any good ideas about what to do with my life, I moved a couple hundred miles away, to a deserted beach town in the middle of winter.

But at least I had "the Dan" to keep me company. I played their first seven albums over and over as I drove up and down the Cape Cod peninsula, searching endlessly for jobs, friends, and places to live. I wanted anything that might provide me with an exciting new direction for myself.

As anyone who's taken what's known as a *geographic cure* knows, though, wherever you go in the world, no matter how amazing, and whoever you find yourself with, no matter how cool, you're still you.

And *you can't hide from what's inside of you*, to quote one of my favorite Steely Dan songs.

The next few years found me hopscotching from one impulsive life decision to the next. I fervently believed that each new career move or change of scene — even getting married and having children — would somehow help me find myself. I wanted something that would make me feel more like me. But also, completely different from the me I was currently living as. Because I wasn't very happy being me.

Long after my party girl days were over, I was still drinking, still drugging, still fantasizing about being someone else, still cutting myself off from anyone who might see the real me, and still trying like hell to escape myself completely. I was more tangled up than I'd ever been. By my early thirties, I found myself in Indiana, of all places, living in a home I hadn't chosen, but which seemed to have been chosen for me.

There was another unpleasant reality that I hadn't chosen, and that I had no idea how to deal with. I could no longer ignore the fact that I was an alcoholic, as well as a drug addict. Nothing I was trying to do on the outside — no character I could become, no cool thing I could get, no world I could inhabit — was making that reality go away.

Not even becoming a freaking addiction therapist!

The great thing about that job, though, is that you can't help but get to know some pretty interesting characters. My first real mentor, a therapist named Kathy, was like a Steely Dan song come to life. Thirty years into her recovery from heroin and alcohol addiction, Kathy may have been small in stature, but she came locked and loaded with an arsenal of life experience.

Kathy was the kind of gritty, witty person who could turn a story about pulling a gun on her abusive ex-husband into a coherent explanation of the cycle of codependency. And she happened to be the first person who saw straight through my glossy surface of high-functionality, to tell me exactly what I needed.

Recovery.

Because it wouldn't be enough just to get sober. *Sobriety*, as Kathy would say, *is just the foundation*. The starting point to finding the real me. The me I'd been burying, numbing, and rebelling against for as long as I could remember. The me who was hurting, scared, and so, so lonely.

But also, according to Kathy, the me who could find healing, belonging, and even self-acceptance. That is, if she could get over herself long enough to accept the help of other recovering people.

Like the fortunate among us addicts, I got the gift of desperation. That desperation drove me to take the help that was offered to me by a Twelve Step fellowship for alcoholics. I was grateful to be accepted and welcomed into its fold, and I ran with it.

But in those first couple years of my recovery, I also ran from staying too long at any one meeting, with any one group of people. I'd stick around a few weeks or months, then get annoyed with some person or another. I told myself that I'd get really serious about the work of recovery when I found the perfect meeting. In the perfect place. At the perfect time. Or with the perfect sponsor.

Until something happened that I would have never predicted. I fell in love.

It was a Monday, of all days, and I'd decided to check out a new meeting. I was walking in circles around a big brick church, trying every door I could see, but finding every one locked. *It's almost like they want me to get drunk tonight*, I thought, cursing whatever jerks were purposely hiding this meeting from me.

I was about to give up and drive away. But on the way back to my car, I ran into someone who could help. It was a priest, of all people. I asked him if he knew where the meeting was, and he led me to a door tucked back in a far corner of the parking lot.

From there, I faced a staircase, and two choices: up or down? I chose down, being the subversive that I am, and found myself in a darkened hallway, where just one room was lit. It turned out to be a middle school classroom.

And that, of all places, was where I fell in love.

Poster boards from a science fair were displayed in one corner, and books I hadn't seen since eighth grade English sat lined up on a table. *Hatchet. Bridge to Terabithia*. And my all-time favorite, *The Wind in the Willows*.

Inspirational quotes lined the walls. *Be yourself! Everyone else is already taken.*

This was the kind of stuff I could imagine my too-cool-for-school, eighth-grade self rolling her eyes at. Now, I just smiled.

I hadn't always liked school. Except there was one year, sixth grade, that I'd loved. I remembered a tiny basement classroom, tucked safely away from the hustle and chaos of the rest of the school. There were ten desks arranged in a neat little circle, and a tall, imposing teacher named Mr. Synnestvedt. As challenging as he was, we knew he expected the best from us, and he always believed we could deliver.

The classroom I found myself in now was like a portal back in time, back when things were simple. Safe. Innocent. And somehow, kind. It was like going back to a time when my future seemed vast and unknown. But also, wide open.

So I guess it was nostalgia that hit me hardest in those first lovestruck moments in that basement classroom. But along with that, I sensed the presence of something even better.

Hope.

Everyone at the meeting was clustered around a group of desks that had been pushed together. It looked like there was no room around that makeshift table, so instinctively I backed away, looking for a seat on the periphery.

Until I heard the old, familiar sound of metal chairs scraping on linoleum.

"Come on over," someone said. "We'll make room."

So I came on over. There was no one I really knew at that meeting. They were talking about a book I'd never really understood, which was full of stories I'd never really read. But if you've ever fallen in love, you'll understand that when love tells you to act, you don't ask too many questions.

That day, love was telling me to stay.

Love was telling me to listen.

Love was telling me to stick with that group of people, in that jumbled basement classroom, and to keep coming back, every Monday night.

Love was telling me to humble myself to let them help me.

And love was telling me that there might be some way I could help them, too.

That process only sounds complicated. But it was pretty simple, the way love did all that. All we had to do was tell stories. We'd start out by reading the ones out of that big blue book, and finish by telling each other stories from our own lives. What we used to be like, in our alcoholism. What happened that got us into recovery. And what our lives were like now.

We told the stories that were a part of us, and always would be. Stories where we'd been the drug dealers. The con men. The disgraced women. And sometimes, the shameless lotharios. I'll admit, though, that I've yet to hear a story in a meeting about being the neighborhood pornographer.

The stories I hear in that meeting — from real, human people, who I've come to consider the closest group of friends I've ever had — are what help me understand myself: a real, human person, too. By getting together every week and sharing our stories, those people have helped me find forgiveness for the mistakes I've made. They also give me hope for the person I want to become.

That meeting is the one place I go every week where I'm guaranteed to feel good — not lost, or confused, or afraid, or insecure. I can get there early and make coffee. I can bring fun-size candy bars. I can set up the chairs and pass out the books. I can greet everyone who walks in, both old-timers and newcomers. I can initiate conversations before the meeting starts.

Those are simple things, but they make me feel like a good person. Better, actually. When I'm at that meeting, I get to be the good person I now know I am.

Who I am, it turns out, has nothing at all to do with what I look like, what I do, or even what my past was. At that meeting, nobody cares that I'm from the East Coast. Nobody cares that I spent my twenties trying to be a professional cool person. Nobody cares that I'm a divorced single mom. Nobody cares that I'm an addiction therapist.

Their love is unconditional: what they care about is *me*.

I've heard a million different ways to describe what love feels like, but the way I experience it is that it makes me feel whole. Secure. Like I've finally come home to myself. And that's exactly what my Monday night home group does for me. It's given me a place where I belong.

I no longer drive around in circles by myself anymore, searching for something that doesn't really exist, anyway. The Unconditional Love I get from my home group has helped me stop hiding from myself, because now I know how good it feels to show myself, and bring out all the love inside me. That love feels like magic, for the way it's transformed me, and for the way I've seen it transform those around me, too.

I can tell you all day long how magical Unconditional Love feels for me, but it won't mean much until you start experiencing it for yourself. Which leads me to the only thing I really know for sure about love.

The more you believe in it, the more you'll start to feel it.

CHAPTER 19

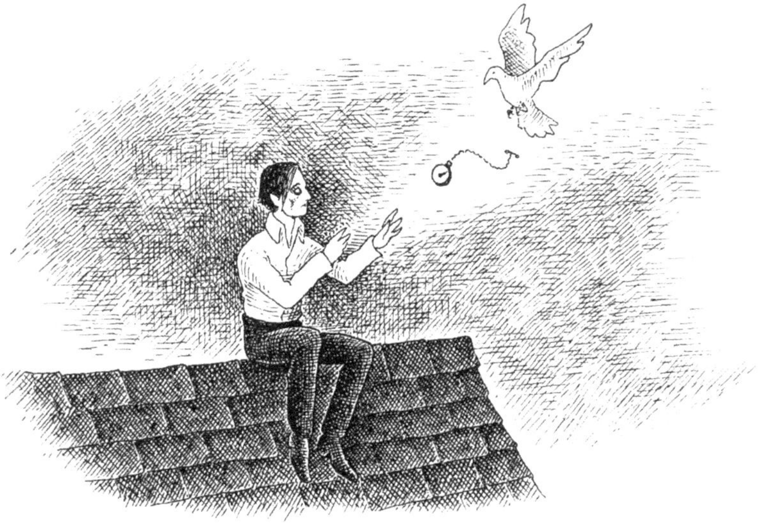

To Believe or Not to Believe

My dear Addict friends, we all have to believe in something. In the same way that a computer's programming determines how it functions, your beliefs determine how you think, how you feel, and how you behave. Even believing in nothing is its own kind of belief. It's just that believing in nothing would mean wandering around life with no rhyme or reason, bumping into walls like a Roomba on the fritz.

Sound familiar?

As humans, we have beliefs about ourselves, beliefs about other people, and beliefs about the way the world works. Beliefs give us security, because we trust them to give us a solid basis for thinking, feeling, and acting. I mean, what else would we trust but *the truth*, as we see it?

Unfortunately, not all beliefs are equally trustworthy, meaning that not all beliefs are true. And when we think, feel, and act on the basis of false beliefs, all bets are off. In fact, holding false beliefs about yourself — such as, *I suck*, or, *I'm inadequate,* or, *I can't handle my problems* —is what made you vulnerable to the manipulative influence of that con artist, Your Addict.

What I've observed, both as an addiction therapist and as a member of my own recovery community, is that no matter who we are or where we come from, addicts hold quite a few false beliefs that have to be completely reprogrammed in recovery. Case in point: our belief in the power of our drug to make us feel good — or at least, better than we did without it. That belief wasn't really about the power of your drug, though.

It was about you.

Believing in your drug means you don't trust the truth

that *you are okay, just as you are*. Instead, you trust the (false) belief that your drug is what makes you okay. And we all know how that turned out: decidedly not okay.

Early sobriety feels particularly awful because when your drug is gone, you're left with unmitigated, unmedicated *fear*. What you're most afraid of, in those first few days, weeks, and months without your drug, is yet another (false) belief: that you no longer have the power to make yourself feel okay.

Talk about feeling powerless!

The biggest problem with getting sober without recovery is that sobriety alone won't help you feel okay — that is, secure — within yourself. True, staying sober is an essential foundation that will go a long way toward getting you back on your feet. But sobriety alone won't challenge your most powerful fear: the deep-seated belief that *you are not okay*.

Recovery is the process of coming to believe that *you are okay, just as you are* — which is another way of saying that recovery is the process of learning to love yourself unconditionally.

And love is the most primal feeling of security there is.

Think of the most powerless kind of human: an infant. Babies literally cry out for love. They need to be held, to be fed and changed, and to have their frenzied, nameless fears gently soothed away. Even when we grow up to be big, strong, complicated adults, feeling loved and cared for is still the most convincing evidence we have for believing the truth that *you are okay, just as you are.*

Yet so many of us addicts have self-identified trust issues when it comes to love. We've been burned. Traumatized. We've had our boundaries trampled on. We've been judged, abandoned, rejected, cheated on, and lied to. All that pain can make the notion of love feel like anything but security.

Other people are inherently unpredictable, I'll give you that. But you can always decide to believe in Unconditional Love for yourself — no matter what. That's part of what makes it unconditional!

Let me say that again. *You have a choice to love yourself, no matter what.*

It's the choice that makes all the difference in determining whether you grow and bloom into Your True Self, or shrink back into the chilly embrace of Your Addict.

Believing that *you are not okay* breeds dishonest relationships filled with anxiety and self-loathing — especially, your relationship with yourself. Believing that *you are okay, just as you are* fosters loving relationships built on honesty, forgiveness, and acceptance — especially, your relationship with yourself.

Look, I don't want to oversimplify the choices and challenges of recovery. All I know is that the longer I walk this road myself, the clearer those choices become.

I can believe in my fears that I'm not okay, and plod

along the same dismal, dead-end road I walked for decades. Or I can trust the Unconditional Love that tells me, *I am okay, just as I am,* and follow a road of limitless rewards that somehow seem as surprising as they are inevitable.

My dear Addict friends, I told you at the outset of this book that recovery is the process of learning how to love. Now I'm going to state what I believe is the truth: that Unconditional Love is the only thing real and powerful enough to help you overcome the fear and shame that fed Your Addict. Unconditional Love is what liberates Your True Self—transforming your life into one of peace, freedom, and happiness.

I can say that all day long, and regale you with all kinds of totally true evidence to back it up. But your recovery depends on whether you believe it's true, too.

I also know that personal experience is the only way you'll come to believe in Unconditional Love. That's why I don't expect you to leap up after reading this book, shouting, *yes, yes, yes! I believe in the power of Unconditional Love!* as you toss your hat into the sky. Believing in *yes* is a choice that only you can make.

But I'd like to point out that even if you don't exactly believe in *yes* right now, you can also choose not to believe in *no*.

No is the language of Your Addict, that self-centered beast who wants to cut you off from connection, and any potential expansion of the love-starved True Self inside you. Your Addict prefers you sitting in a big stinking puddle of fear and shame, where you will circle the drain of drugs, disconnection, and self-destruction in an attempt to numb your need for love.

Believing only in *no* means you will see only phonies and hypocrites at play in the recovery meeting rooms I've described, instead of acceptance and hope at work. Believing only in *no* means you are destined to ditch the ideas in this book, and go searching for the solution to Your Addict problem in another pill or another doctor, instead. Believing only in *no* means you will try to find security in a person, place, or thing, instead of finding ways to connect to the Unconditional Love that already lies at the heart of you.

My dear Addict friends, if you find yourself rejecting the solution of recovery, and all it consists of — the process of getting sober, the rigorous honesty, the connection with other recovering addicts, and the call to believe in something bigger and more powerful than your drug — I think you have to ask yourself one fundamental question.

Do I really know better, on my own — or am I just afraid of what I don't yet know?

Please don't disown or deny that fear. Let yourself see the truth of it, and be honest about it. And let the power of your truth — rather than the power of your fear —

guide you on your next steps toward uncovering more and more truth about yourself.

Every single statement of personal truth that you can make, whether you consider it good, bad, or ugly, is a step toward practicing Unconditional Love for Your True Self.

CHAPTER 20

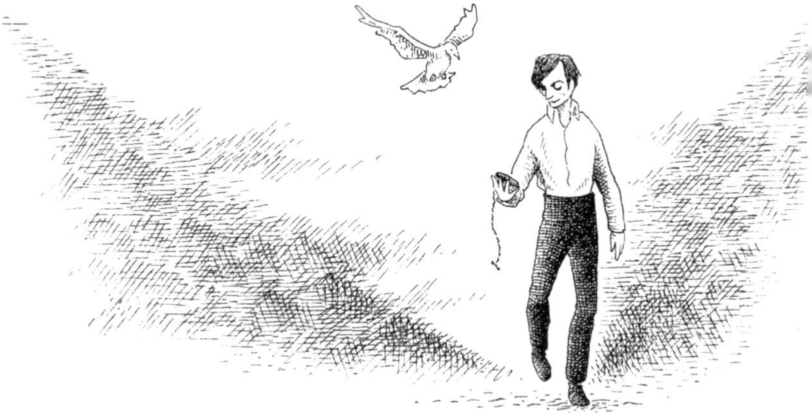

Good Orderly Direction

My own recovery began with a head-on collision with fear.

Those fears hit me in the form of paralyzing panic attacks, following my separation from my ex-husband. I was a therapist in training then, trying to keep it together while hanging on by my fingernails to the roller coaster ride that is divorce. With my career and the prospect of single-motherhood at stake, I was terrified of my feelings taking control of me at any given moment. I was also trying to stop drinking, so I didn't even have alcohol to numb the intensity of my anxiety, anger, and depression.

I felt helpless to help myself, until a kind-hearted neighbor plucked me out of my emotional exile and brought me to my first meeting for recovering alcoholics.

Humbling myself in those rooms of recovery as someone who needed to be helped, rather than positioning myself as the helper, wasn't the humiliating experience I'd imagined it would be. Instead, it was like coming upon a cold, clear pool of water after wandering through the desert for several decades. I had no idea I was so thirsty for acceptance and understanding.

The first thing that happened was that all the painful feelings I'd been hiding inside came tumbling out in a torrent of tears. I was so grateful for the three minutes a week I could pour my heart out to those lovely, understanding strangers. I came to look forward to those meetings so much, I wildly overpaid my babysitter to ensure I'd never miss them.

Being in the midst of a divorce, I wasn't exactly pondering the nature of Unconditional Love back then. Yet I could feel the sobriety-sustaining power of love every time I walked into those meeting rooms. Anyone could tell their story of alcoholic insanity and be accepted.

Everyone was given the chance to speak honestly, without interruption or opposition. And everyone was given the same opportunity for recovery. Absolutely no one was denied hope.

My first sponsor in that program was a woman I was drawn to because she had a palpable glow about her. She was joyful. Exuberant. Liberated. Monica, as I'll call her, had been in recovery for several years. And that inner radiance was exactly what I wanted, even if I didn't know what it was about just yet.

It didn't take me long to realize that Monica was what you might call a "God lady." Not a *praise Jesus!* type, as she never discussed the nature of her belief system. But she certainly wasn't shy about telling me how her faith in the power of God had restored her alcoholic life to a sane one in sobriety.

Rather than pushing her own beliefs on me, Monica simply encouraged me to acknowledge the mysterious and benevolent process that was unfolding in my first few months of recovery.

"First, you come," Monica would say, about the necessity of getting to meetings regularly. "Then, you come to," she'd say, about accepting the reality of my alcoholism, and that there was hope for my recovery.

"And then," she'd say, beaming, "you come to believe."

That last part, I was a little shaky on. "Believe in... what, exactly? Who?"

"It's okay," Monica would tell me. "You don't have to know right now. Stick around, you'll figure it out."

I'd never had a God in my life, and I certainly didn't believe in one. My parents were atheists, so I'd grown up without any religious or spiritual beliefs whatsoever. I'd say I was an atheist, too, but the truth was, I'd never really thought about God long enough to have any beliefs about its existence, or lack thereof.

As far as love and security were concerned, I had believed so hard, and for so long, in the power of drugs and alcohol to bring me comfort. Beyond that, I believed only in my own powers of reason and intelligence to make decisions.

But something wasn't adding up there, anymore. There was no comfort or security left in drugs and alcohol. They only made me feel sick and ashamed of myself. Yet I kept trusting them to take care of me, which was completely unreasonable, and utterly lacking in intelligence. The world inside my head was swirling with fear, and I was an emotional wreck to prove it.

It was clear that I needed something more solid to live by than my usual cesspool of anxious thoughts, painful feelings, and self-sabotaging behavior. Call it the gift of desperation, but I began listening to Monica talk about the role of God in her recovery with an open mind — or maybe, bewildered fascination was more like it.

Ever the apt pupil, I had the *why* of God figured out

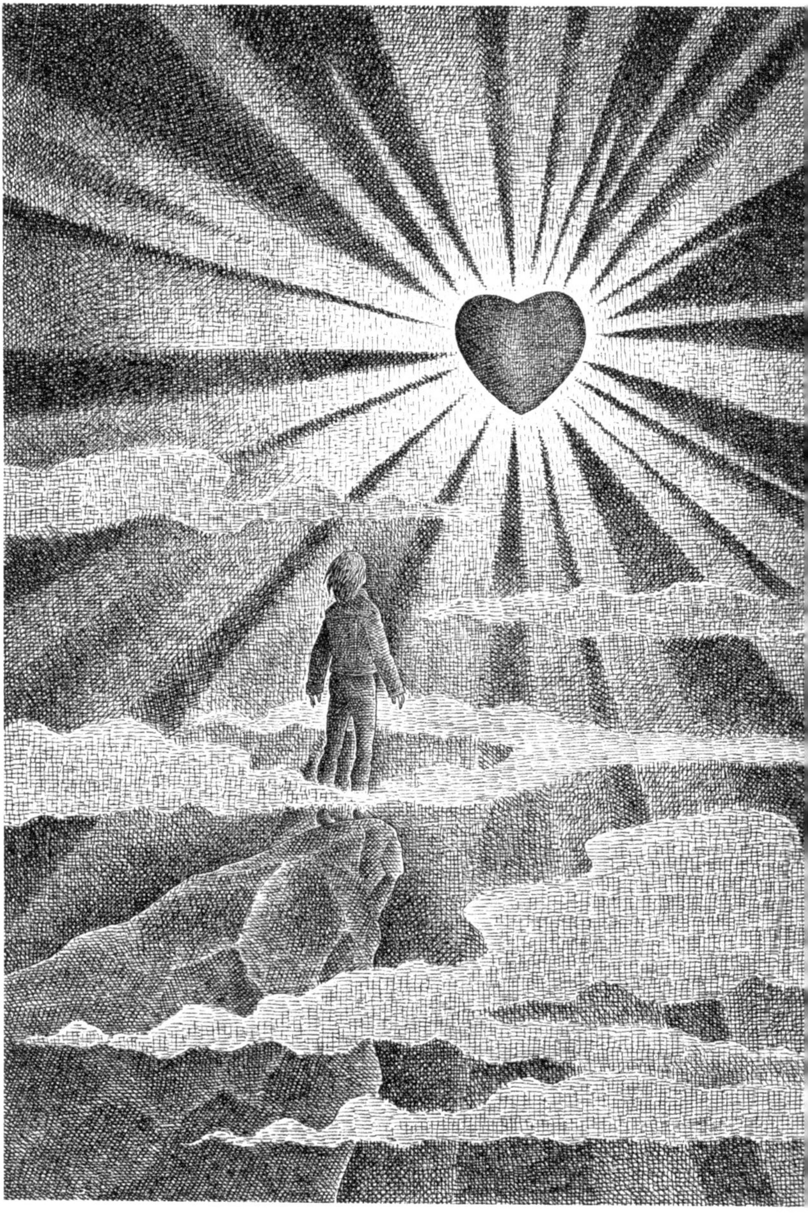

long before the *how*. I knew I needed values to anchor me. I needed a source of meaning to inspire me. I needed comfort when I felt broken, and I needed guidance when I felt lost.

Monica gave me an acronym that helped keep it simple, as well as secular.

"Just think of God as Good, Orderly Direction," she said. "Good, because it's a loving presence in your life. Orderly, to give you a solid basis to make decisions. And direction, which will move you forward."

When it came to believing in the Good, Orderly Direction of God — or, in the language of that recovery fellowship, *a power greater than myself* — I couldn't argue with the evidence around me. The recovering alcoholics in those meetings were staying sober on the basis of their belief in something more powerful than their drug. They were loving, they were honest, and they were hopeful, which seemed like a far better basis for living than anything I was coming up with on my own.

I was getting the gist of this God thing. But I still needed something more solid. I couldn't bring myself to just believe in — let alone pray or meditate to — an empty space I couldn't see. That made me feel more alone than ever.

What I needed was a face. Even better? A pretty face.

Here's where it gets a little weird, my dear Addict friends. But it goes to show that where there's a will, there's a way. Especially when it comes to your willingness to believe in the truth.

Besides those recovery meetings, the only other thing that was getting me through the darkness of my divorce was '80s music. My True Self has always loved '80s music, going all the way back to my '80s childhood. To keep myself from crying and drinking at night, I started a blog where I wrote album reviews and fan fiction about the New Romantics.

The New Romantics were a wave of bands from Britain in the early '80s. They wore poufy shirts, sported great hair, and wrote even greater love songs. One of my favorites was a band called Spandau Ballet, a group of five guys who had impeccable style and albums with a lot of heart.

Spandau Ballet's lead singer was a heartthrob named Tony Hadley. Dark, debonair Tony Hadley. Tony Hadley of the three-piece suits and gold pinky rings. Tony Hadley, who had a voice that could melt butter, and a face that melted millions of teenage girls' hearts. Tony Hadley, who reminded me of my long ago, bright-eyed innocence. Tony Hadley, who seemed to know so much about love, and whose voice inspired so many feelings of love in my heart.

Love was what I was seeing and experiencing in those recovery meetings, and love was the Good, Orderly Direction I wanted to guide my life, even if I didn't know what that would look like yet. But as far as looks went, Tony

Hadley was the undisputed '80s embodiment of love. That made him an ideal — if unlikely — figurehead for my own working concept of God.

So I started a little dialogue with myself that first year of my recovery, that year I was searching for an understanding of a power greater than myself. Instead of, *what would Jesus do?* I began to ask myself, *what would Tony Hadley do?*

Tony Hadley would be kind, of course. Generous. He would be self-aware enough to accept his feelings, and he would be understanding of the feelings of others. If there was a conflict, he would gallantly offer to be the bigger person. And though an obstacle or a rejection might darken his mood for a moment, Tony Hadley would be the last person to throw a cell phone, let alone go on a three-day booze binge.

Above all, Tony Hadley would be honest. After all, Spandau's biggest hit was a song called "True."

I had no illusions about Tony Hadley actually being God, but it was a reliably appealing way for My True Self to start orienting my thoughts, feelings, and actions toward love. At the very least, imagining *what would Tony Hadley do?* made me giggle, and it gave me hope that I could bring the fierce and undying love I had for Spandau Ballet to other parts of my life, too.

My belief in the power of love strengthened and solidified over the next couple of years, as I kept attending those recovery meetings for alcoholics. I had stopped drinking, I was healing my wounds in the care of people who understood me, and I was making friends — real friends. These were people I was happy to see every week, who seemed genuinely happy to see me, too. I was letting them get to know me, as I shared more about how alcohol had screwed up so many of my opportunities and relationships.

I felt accepted. I felt inspired by the hope those recovering alcoholics had for me. And I felt loved, at least, to the extent that I was willing to practice Unconditional Love. But at the end of the day, I wasn't being honest about the fact that I was still going home and smoking tons of weed.

It didn't make sense, even to me. I had all these supportive, sober friends. I had a sponsor I could trust. I was immersed in the culture of recovery, both in my own meetings and in my therapy practice with recovering addicts. I had even come to believe in the power of Unconditional Love.

But I couldn't let go of the fear that I wouldn't be okay if I didn't have at least one way left to get high.

Think of a child's most basic fear: being alone in the dark. I was afraid of that, too. I was afraid to give up the drug I believed in, in spite of all the ways it had betrayed me and stolen my freedom. I was afraid of the vast, unknown darkness I might face in its absence.

But at a certain point, I began to feel more desperate than afraid.

It's often said that necessity is the mother of invention. I'll go one further, offering that desperation is the mother of rebirth and transformation. A desperate addict understands the truth that their way of living no longer means life. That was true for me, toward the end of using my drug. I was facing too much darkness, the way I was going. I could no longer believe that I knew better, alone in my miserable cell of secrecy and shame.

But it wasn't just intellectually believing in the power of love that was going to help me get sober, after relying for so long on some drug or another to take care of my fears. After all, I'd just spent my first few years in recovery sitting on my yoga mat and smoking weed, kidding myself that getting high while meditating on the concept of love made me feel closer to love than ever. Meanwhile, I hated myself for using that drug, which was counterproductive to fostering self-love — to say the least.

No, I had to start acting like I believed in Unconditional Love. Following Good, Orderly Direction meant being honest, no matter how hard it was.

First, I had to tell the truth to my honesty coach, by reaching out to him for help and admitting that I was powerless over my drug. Then, I had to go to online meetings for recovering marijuana addicts, which was pretty much the only place where anyone would take me seriously when I told them how much pain my weed addiction was causing me.

There were so. Many. Meetings. I went once, twice, and sometimes three times a day — whenever I started getting restless, irritable, and discontent, or whenever a craving threatened to overtake me.

Without a doubt, making the decision to be sober from weed, *right now*, was my biggest-ever leap of faith in the name of Good, Orderly Direction. It was the true test of my belief in Unconditional Love: that *I am okay, just as I am.*

All that truth-telling was hard, but the hardest part was telling the truth to you, my dear Addict friends. Eventually, I had to come clean to the listeners of my recovery podcast, which included some of my therapy clients. I had to admit that their so-called recovery evangelist had been living the double life of an addict, up until very recently.

Ah, yes. I was still smoking weed and living as My Addict for the first nine months I was writing and podcasting — wait for it — this book about recovery. My Addict justified it by telling me that weed helped me be more creative. It even told me that continuing to suffer in my addiction would help me authentically connect with the still-suffering addict I was writing for. Not that I dared to be transparent about My Addict's brilliant plan while I was still using my drug, of course.

It was about a year into my weed sobriety that I began to take those first steps toward honesty on the podcast. Chapter by chapter, I told my dear Addict friends the story of my sick, sad weed addiction, and how much damage it had done to me. At the risk of discrediting myself as a recovery evangelist, not to mention losing my day job as an addiction therapist, I also told them how recently I had gotten sober.

I took that risk of honesty because I believed in its value to other recovering addicts who were trying to get honest, too.

I took that risk of honesty because I believed it was an act of Unconditional Love for My True Self.

And I took that risk of honesty because I had faith that following the road of Unconditional Love would lead me to my greatest good.

It did. Among other rewards — like all the support and encouragement I got from my recovery community — that honesty made me feel lighter. Freer. Giddy, even. Like I was dancing around in the outrageously sunny light of true self-acceptance.

After that big reveal, though, I did what addicts do: I went overboard. All hyped up on my newfound sobriety, I started trying to control other people's, too. Both in my therapy office and on the podcast, I tried to tell everyone to do the same things that had worked for me. I tried to tell them exactly which drugs they needed to be sober from. And I tried to push their fears away before they were ready to let go of them, themselves.

In other words, I made other people's recovery all about me.

By selling a particular agenda instead of simply providing acceptance and hope, I was putting conditions on what should have been unconditional: the love I was trying to help them foster for their own True Selves. Oops.

Soon enough, I got humbled. About two years into my weed sobriety, I relapsed. Who knew that THC gummies were just as addictive as smoking, vaping, or dabbing weed? Answer: *me*.

Before I used again, I knew the truth that I'd still be powerless. I knew it would bring back all the old fear and shame My Addict thrived so hard on. And I knew it was going to suck to have to get sober all over again. But I used anyway. And that's the truth.

This time, though, I was honest about it immediately, with anyone who would listen. And I'm still telling the truth about it. Not just here in this book, but also with my clients (when they inquire), at my recovery meetings, and on the podcast, where I've narrated my journey back to sobriety.

Maybe some people think it's professional suicide to admit I've been anything other than a perfect, sober superhero. But for anyone who cares to hear the truth, I care to share my true life experience. That's because I believe that hiding in shame will keep me sick, while being honest in the name of Unconditional Love will get me… well, I have no idea, really!

I may not know where I'll end up, but I have faith that practicing honesty will continue to lead me to my greatest good. I also know that I feel peace, freedom, and happiness when I believe in the truth that *I am okay, just as I am*. In fact, I'd say that learning to love myself has been the best and biggest reward of taking step after step in that Good, Orderly Direction.

The truth is, I am where I am right now, and I am who I am right now. The fact is, it took what it took to get me to accept the truth about my powerlessness over drugs and alcohol, and to stop using each and every one of them in the order and in the time frame that I did. That includes my last relapse, too.

So who am I to argue with the truth? Why do I think I need to rewrite history? And why would I try to put conditions on the inherently unconditional nature of love? Love, after all, is what I've experienced to be far more powerful and healing than any other therapeutic intervention I've subjected myself to over the years. And as long as I keep doing my best to follow love's benevolent but mysterious path, who am I to say how the process should unfold?

Who's to say that it wasn't the audacious act of trying to do a podcast and write a book about recovery —

beginning when I wasn't sober — that helped me accept the truth about how badly I needed to get sober?

My dear Addict friends, for most of you, recovery will feel like the first chance you've had at learning to love Your True Self. At least, since you were brand new to the world, back before you lost your innocence. Before you decided you needed to do, or to be, or to act a certain way to be okay. Before you felt you came up short on those counts, and started hiding.

As long as you stay committed to recovering, uncovering, and discovering Your True Self, you've got the chance to launch yourself into a whole new realm of existence. Just like we were all forced to do, as newborn babes evicted from the cramped darkness of our mother's womb.

And just like a real birth, it's gonna take a minute to rub the goo out of your eyes. You're gonna wriggle and grunt and tell everyone you know that you can't do it, it's too hard, you want to go back. You're gonna scream and cry and maybe even wet your pants a little.

That's fine. Go ahead and scream! Release all the fear inside you by letting out a long, shuddering cry for help, just like you did in your first moments of existence. Something in you then trusted that something out there would take care of you. And it did, didn't it? You're here now, aren't you?

If you can muster up enough honesty to let your cry for help be known, I promise that Unconditional Love will fall all over itself to help you. It's got an infinite number of ingenious ways to reward your fledgling trust in the truth. The most important thing is that you emerge from your hiding place of shame with Your Addict's hands up.

Call it desperation. Call it baptism by fire. But I call this massively courageous act of giving yourself up and turning yourself over to the light *surrender.*

So if there are any miserable addicts reading this, I say to you, *surrender, already.* Take the hand offered to you by recovery, and step away from the ruins left behind by your drug. Surrendering to the solution of recovery means you are isolated and hopeless no more. No longer is Your True Self condemned to diminish and die in the prison of Your Addict's fear and shame.

In this case, surrender means freedom — not defeat.

As you learn to love, and your journey into the heart of Your True Self gets deeper and deeper, it won't be a matter of hope, or even mere trust, anymore. You'll be building faith that you're being taken care of by Good, Orderly Direction, because you'll feel the touch of love.

Love, my dear Addict friends, feels like peace. Freedom. And happiness.

Not to worry. It'll all make sense soon enough. The truth has a funny way of doing that.

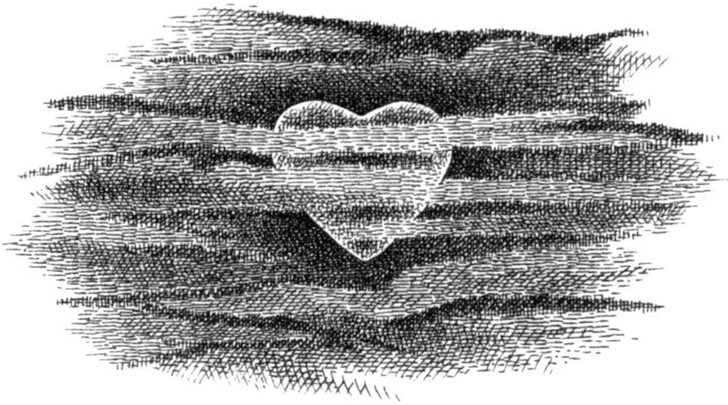

PREVIEW OF BOOK TWO

The Addict's Guide to Love

Where we left off, my dear Addict friends, you were screaming for help. A gigantic primal scream that reverberated into the farthest reaches of the universe.

A scream that said nothing, but expressed everything. Fear. Regret. Humiliation. Anger. Disbelief, even, that the illusion of security you've been clinging to all this time turned out to be a hoax.

Those walls you spent a lifetime building — and all the self-reliance and mistrust that fortified them — only ended up imprisoning you in a lonely castle of fear. How cruel was the irony that your fear of pain and suffering was so much of what was causing your pain and suffering!

So go ahead. Keep screaming. It's your birthright to rebel against a life of pain and suffering, no matter how you got here. Let your rebel yell of protest be known. Because it's not the truth that hurts you, it's the lies you've been living.

You don't have to live like that anymore.

Maybe you're beginning to sense that too. So maybe, just maybe, that scream wasn't all panic and desperation. Maybe, amidst the fear, the regret, the humiliation, and the anger, there was relief in that scream. Anticipation. Even an emerging sense of awe.

Because maybe you're beginning to believe me when I tell you that all the worst things you've ever believed about yourself — all your so-called deficiencies and limitations, and all your hopelessness about the world around you — aren't actually the truth. Maybe the idea of the universe being a loving, caring place gives you hope, even if you can't quite bring yourself to believe that it's the truth quite yet.

And so maybe, just maybe, that gigantic scream signals that you're willing to make this utterly unknown journey into truth for yourself. There's a little voice inside you that's dying to know if all this crazy Unconditional Love stuff turns out to be true.

Who knows? Maybe you'll come to love the way you look and feel in the truth.

But what now? What happens after the scream?

I'm not going to sugarcoat it, folks. You're just waking up to an entirely new level of consciousness. Not in your comfortable bed, I might add, but somewhere completely unknown.

The first thing you feel, upon awakening, is the unforgivingly solid ground beneath you. Your head feels thick, your mouth is parched, and when you try to open your eyes, you find they're nearly swollen shut. Your muscles ache, as though your whole body has been wrenched and thrown about. It's like you're regaining consciousness after some major trauma. Was there an accident? A plane crash? It takes enormous effort to sit upright as you lean back, gingerly, on your palms.

Where are you?

You feel it before you know it: the unmistakable effects of a high noon sun in a cloudless sky. White light burns the insides of your eyelids. Your face grows hot. Sound is absent, save for the cry of birds that echoes in the stillness of your surroundings.

You are outside.
Somewhere.
Outside.

You blink as hard as you can, until what's around you starts to come into focus. That sun is everywhere. Not just up high, but also glinting relentlessly off the lake that surrounds you. You see the deep greens of trees — not the stubby trees of suburbia, but the enormous rugged trees of the wilderness. They tower over you, in silent command of the natural landscape that stretches out so, so far beyond you.

You sit up straighter, blink harder. You can feel tears forming at the corners of your eyes.

You are outside.
In an unknown wilderness.
And you are utterly alone.

This cannot be. But it is! You are not dreaming. You, a comfortable child — of the city, the suburbs, or even the countryside — are no match for this untamed wilderness. Nothing that you know is here. There's no trace of the stuff that has constituted your daily life and ensured your survival up until now.

No homes. No stores. No phones. No electricity, no cars, no maps, no clothes, no job, no money. No cover. No protection.

Your tears are flowing freely now, stinging the wounded flesh of your cheeks.

It occurs to you that you have no identity out here, no past that's relevant to anything in these surroundings. The birds — do they give one single fuck who you are?

You yourself know only one thing at this moment: that whatever your life is about to become, it's going to be between you and nature.

I'll remind you now, though, that you are not alone.

This new phase of your life is not about you versus nature — or you against the world, for that matter. It's about you getting closer to nature: your true nature. You, my dear Addict friend, are an essential part of a beautiful universe that is infinitely capable of loving and caring for Your True Self.

That is, as long as you're up for the challenge of learning to trust it, instead of letting yourself slip back into hiding and being afraid of it. But I know how terrifying it is to surrender everything you know and take the great leap of faith that is trust.

Universal trust, no less.

Think of it this way, though — what else are you going to trust out here? Your tired old collection of nameless fears, distorted beliefs, and insufferable self-loathing? How are those supposed to further your survival in the natural world, which refuses to be manipulated into taking pity on you, in the face of those lies?

Indeed, you're at that awkward point in your recovery where you can at least trust the truth that there are no alternatives to living in the truth!

I'll admit that I often wish, somewhat perversely, that everyone I work with in early recovery would find themselves in the metaphorical circumstances I'm describing here. Stranded in the wilderness with their slate wiped utterly clean, all their emotional crutches and illusions of safety gone. They'd be armed with nothing but pure feeling, acute awareness, and the will to live.

Recovery boot camp, indeed.

Think of how quickly it would become clear that fear was a luxury you could no longer afford. Instead, your most precious resource would be *trust*. And not only trust in nature to provide for you. As part of that, you would have to trust yourself — to learn how to harmonize with and harness the natural world around you.

As a matter of fact, trust would be the only thing you could do, aside from lay down and die.

But first things first. I don't want to minimize the pain and confusion you're experiencing, as you stand here today on the precipice of such a drastic change in consciousness. You are injured, disoriented, and scared shitless. What a painfully rude awakening you were met with at the dawn of this new era!

As uncomfortable and uncertain as you feel right now, though, I want you to think back to that unacceptable state of affairs that prompted you to let out that enormous scream. You may have been sober, but you were still crawling out of your own skin with the same old hurts, fears, and hangups you've always had.

That was what thrust you into this decision to face

everything and recover — to recover your truth. To do nothing would be to allow Your Addict to seduce you back into a complete obliteration of Your True Self.

So here you are, lurching toward that ultimate truth, destination unknown, with the only truth you do know to guide your way. The good news is that that's enough. It's time to stop looking outside yourself for your sense of security and self-worth. It's time to stop relying on any particular person, place, or thing, or to any particular set of circumstances, to tell you that *you are okay, just as you are.*

Instead, you will learn to trust the natural laws of the universe to bring you the security and the good you've always longed for. That means bringing the only things you truly can control — your thoughts, your feelings, and your actions — into harmony with those universal laws.

One step at a time, in the chapters that follow, you will learn about the process of applying this trust, like a thick coat of love, to every element of your own universe. To your present life, of course, but also to your past, to your future, to your relationships, to your purpose, and to the greater world around you.

Take heart, my dear Addict friends. By screaming out loud how much you need this love and strength, you're already heading in the right direction: toward truth, truth, and nothing but the truth.

In other words, you're exactly where you need to be right now.

RESOURCES

Disclaimer: The information about these free, mutual-aid recovery support groups and resources has been adapted from the mission statements and information available on each organization's website. Inclusion on this list does not necessarily represent the views or endorsement of the author. Please also note that individuals who are at risk for moderate to severe withdrawal symptoms should consult a medical professional before beginning a program of recovery.

Alcoholics Anonymous
aa.org
Offers in-person and online meetings

Alcoholics Anonymous is a fellowship of men and women who share their experience, strength, and hope with each other, so they may solve their common problem and help others recover from alcoholism. The only requirement is a desire to stop drinking. AA is not allied with any sect, denomination, politics, organization, or institution. Its primary purpose is to help its members stay sober, and help others to achieve sobriety.

Buddhist Recovery Network
buddhistrecovery.org
Offers in-person and online meetings

The Buddhist Recovery Network promotes the use of Buddhist teachings and practices to help people recover from the suffering caused by addictive behaviors. It is open to people of all backgrounds, and it is respectful of all recovery paths.

Celebrate Recovery
celebraterecovery.com
Offers in-person and online meetings

As a Christian-based support group, Celebrate Recovery centers meetings on Christian scripture as a means to find strength during recovery. The recovery model at Celebrate Recovery teaches participants to accept that a higher power is in control. This group also provides support for non-addiction issues, such as depression and low self-esteem.

Cocaine Anonymous
ca.org
Offers in-person and online meetings

Cocaine Anonymous is a fellowship of men and women who share their experience, strength and hope with each other, that they may solve their common problem and help others recover from their addiction. The best way to reach someone is to speak to them on a common level, which is why CA members maintain their individual sobriety by working with others. Members come from various social, ethnic, economic and religious backgrounds, but what they have in common is addiction. Anyone who wants to stop using cocaine and all other mind-altering substances is welcome.

Crystal Meth Anonymous
crystalmeth.org
Offers in-person and online meetings

Crystal Meth Anonymous (CMA) is a fellowship of people who share their experience, strength, and hope with each other, that they may solve their common problem and help others to recover from crystal meth addiction. The only requirement for membership is a desire to stop using. There are no dues or fees for CMA membership; they are self-supporting through their own contributions. CMA is not allied with any religion, sect, denomination, political group, organization, or institution. Its primary purpose is to lead a sober life and to carry the message of recovery to the crystal meth addict who still suffers.

Gamblers Anonymous
gamblersanonymous.org
Offers in-person and online meetings

Gamblers Anonymous (GA) is a fellowship of men and women who share their experience, strength and hope with each other, that they may solve their common problem and help others recover from a gambling problem. The only requirement for membership is a desire to stop gambling. The fellowship's primary purpose is to stop gambling and to help other compulsive gamblers do the same.

Heroin Anonymous
heroinanonymous.org
Offers in-person and online meetings

Heroin Anonymous (HA) is a fellowship of men and women who have found a better way of life, free from heroin addiction. Its fellowship is based on a Twelve Step program of recovery. There are no dues or fees for membership; the only requirement for membership is a desire to stop suffering from heroin addiction. The HA fellowship works to assist the next person seeking help with their own addiction.

Jewish Alcoholics, Chemically Dependent Persons and Significant Others (JACS)
jewishboard.org/listing/jacs-jcsrecovery/

For information about meetings, visit the website or email JCSRecovery@jbfcs.org

JACS is a grassroots, volunteer-driven organization that is committed to self-help and mutual support. JACS members, representing the entire spectrum of Jewish experience, background, affiliation and observance, are able to connect with one another, explore their Jewish roots, and discover resources within Judaism to enhance their recovery.

LifeRing Secular Recovery
lifering.org
Offers in-person and online meetings

LifeRing Secular Recovery is an organization of people who share practical experiences and sobriety support. There are as many ways to live free of illicit or non-medically indicated drugs and alcohol as there are stories of successful sober people, and many LifeRing members attend other recovery programs as well. LifeRing's emphasis on the positive can turn anger and despair into hope and resolve. LifeRing respectfully embraces what works for each individual. Its members share advice, understanding, and encouragement. LifeRing meetings focus primarily on the present, not on the hurts and damages of the past.

Marijuana Anonymous
marijuana-anonymous.org
Offers in-person and online meetings

Marijuana Anonymous is a fellowship of people who share their experience, strength, and hope with one another, to help solve their common problem and help others to recover from marijuana addiction. The only requirement for membership is a desire to stop using marijuana.

Millati Islami
millatiislami.org
Offers in-person and online meetings

Millati Islami is a fellowship of men and women who join together on the "Path of Peace." Members share their experience, strength, and hope while recovering from active addiction to mind and mood-altering substances. Members look to Allah (God) to guide them on Millati Islami (the Path of Peace). They strive to become rightly guided Muslims, submitting their will and services to Allah. The program seeks to integrate the requirements of Al-Islam with the Twelve Step approach to recovery. Millati Islami was born out of its members' need to be religiously specific with regard to spiritual principles.

Narcotics Anonymous
na.org
Offers in-person and online meetings

Narcotics Anonymous (NA) is a global, community-based organization with a multilingual and multicultural membership. It offers recovery from the effects of addiction by means of working a Twelve Step program, including regular attendance at group meetings. The Narcotics Anonymous name is not meant to imply a focus on any particular drug; NA's approach makes no distinction between drugs, including alcohol.

Nicotine Anonymous
nicotine-anonymous.org
Offers in-person and online meetings

Nicotine Anonymous (NicA) is a non-profit Twelve Step fellowship of people helping each other live nicotine-free lives. NicA welcomes all those seeking freedom from nicotine addiction, including those using cessation programs and nicotine withdrawal aids. The primary purpose of NicA is to help all those who would like to cease using tobacco and nicotine products in any form. The Fellowship offers group support and recovery using the Twelve Steps and Twelve Traditions, as adapted from Alcoholics Anonymous, to achieve abstinence from nicotine.

Overeaters Anonymous

oa.org

Offers in-person and online meetings

Overeaters Anonymous (OA) is a community of people who support each other in order to recover from compulsive eating and food behaviors. Its members welcome everyone who feels they have a problem with food.

Pagans in Recovery

pagansinrecovery.org

Offers in-person and online meetings

Pagans in Recovery is a Twelve Step fellowship based on the model pioneered by Alcoholics Anonymous. It aims to give hope to people seeking recovery that they can recover without having to accept anyone else's beliefs, or deny their own. The fellowship welcomes those who worship or work with one or more Goddesses, Gods, Spirits, Energies, Powers, or Ancestors, and whose spirituality may include magical practices. Pagans in Recovery is not specific to any individual Twelve Step program, nor does it wish to compete with or replace them. The fellowship is available to all who need it, to be used in conjunction with more targeted programs that address each person's specific issues. Because of this diversity within its community, Pagans in Recovery defines recovery in multiple ways. As such, the recovery language used in its meetings (for example, "sobriety") is left up to each individual to decide.

Pills Anonymous
pillsanonymous.org
Offers in-person and online meetings

Pills Anonymous is a fellowship of men and women who share their experience, strength, and hope with each other, that they may solve their common problem and help others to recover from pill addiction. The only requirement for membership is a desire to stop using pills. The program works when members regularly attend meetings and work the Twelve Steps of recovery with other pill addicts. The fellowship works together to help its members stay clean and help others achieve the same freedom.

Secular Organizations for Sobriety (SOS)
sossobriety.org
Offers in-person and online meetings

Secular Organizations for Sobriety is a nonprofit network of autonomous, non-professional local groups that are dedicated solely to helping individuals achieve and maintain sobriety/abstinence from alcohol and drug addiction, food addiction, and other types of addiction.

Sex Addicts Anonymous
saa-recovery.org
Offers in-person and online meetings

As a fellowship of recovering addicts, Sex Addicts Anonymous offers a message of hope to anyone who suffers from sex addiction. Through long and painful experience, SAA members came to realize that they were powerless over their sexual thoughts and behaviors, and that their preoccupation with sex was causing progressively severe adverse consequences for themselves, their families, and their friends. Many members came to that realization when they began attending SAA meetings, where they heard stories similar to their own, and realized that recovery was possible. Through the SAA fellowship, members learn that they are not hopelessly defective.

Sex and Love Addicts Anonymous
https://slaafws.org/
Offers in-person and online meetings

Sex and Love Addicts Anonymous (S.L.A.A.) is a program for anyone who suffers from an addictive compulsion to engage in (or avoid) sex, love, or emotional attachment. It uses the Twelve Steps and Twelve Traditions adapted from Alcoholics Anonymous to recover from these compulsions. Its members are united in a common focus: dealing with addictive sexual and emotional behavior. They find a common denominator in obsessive/compulsive patterns, which transcends any personal differences of sexual orientation or gender identity.

SMART Recovery
smartrecovery.org
Offers in-person and online meetings

SMART stands for Self-Management and Recovery Training. It is a transformative method of moving from addictive substances and negative behaviors to a life of positive self-regard and the willingness to change. SMART was created for people seeking a self-empowering way to overcome addictive problems. Peers and professionals working together fuse science and experience to help members build healthy and balanced lives.

Substance Abuse and Mental Health Services Administration (SAMHSA)
https://www.samhsa.gov/find-help/national-helpline

SAMHSA's National Helpline, 1-800-662-HELP (4357) (also known as the Treatment Referral Routing Service), or 1-800-487-4889, is a confidential, free, 24-hour-a-day, 365-day-a-year information service, available in English and Spanish, for individuals and family members facing mental health and/or substance use disorders. This service provides referrals to local treatment facilities, support groups, and community-based organizations. Visit SAMHSA's online treatment locator, or send your zip code via text message to 435748 (HELP4U) to find help near you.

Women For Sobriety (WFS)
womenforsobriety.org
Offers in-person and online meetings

Women for Sobriety (WFS) is an organization whose purpose is to help women find their individual path to recovery through their discovery of self. WFS is an abstinence-based program for women overcoming challenges with alcohol and the use of other drugs. The New Life Program in WFS acknowledges the needs women have in recovery – the need to nurture feelings of self-value and self-worth, and the desire to discard feelings of guilt, shame, and humiliation. WFS is not affiliated with any other recovery organization; it stands on its own principles and philosophies.

ACKNOWLEDGMENTS

In addition to my parents, who have supported and loved me unconditionally since my first day of existence, I have many other people to thank here. Each of them has, in their own way, helped me become the kind of therapist, writer, and human being who could write this book.

Thank you to Dr. Cullen Hardy, for being the honesty coach I needed, at exactly the time I needed one. To my teachers, the late Michael Grinfeld, Mary Smith, and Jared Synnestvedt, for fostering my love of reading and writing. To Kathy Wenger, for showing me the honest way to be an addiction therapist. To John Horsley, for giving me the chance to learn from the pros. To Pat Hancock, for granting me the freedom to build a substance abuse program from the ground up. To Ellen Jones, for helping me through the hardest time of my life. And to Kristin Brandon, for advocating for me through all of my grad school struggles, both real and imagined.

Thank you to my Thursday night "Life After Sobriety" group, for never being afraid to say *I love you.* To my home group crew at the Monday night Big Book meeting at St. Monica's, for always showing up and showing me love. And to Bill W. and Dr. Bob, for being the first to carry the message of recovery.

And then there are my teachers on the page — too many to list, but I'll try. Thank you to Craig Nakken, Brad Blanton, Melody Beattie, Rick Carson, David G. Benner, Patrick Carnes, John A. Sanford, Irvin Yalom, John Powell, and Michael A. Singer, for writing with such grace and wisdom about addiction, recovery, therapy, and spirituality. To Robert Greene, for showing me what's possible with ambition, wit, and inspiration. To Florence Shinn, Ernest Holmes, Jen Sincero, and Rhonda Byrne, for giving me the gift of faith in my own vision. To Gary Paulsen, Roald Dahl, Mary Gaitskill, Rosamunde Pilcher, Iris Murdoch, and scores of other fiction writers whose gifts for storytelling swept me off my feet, and to Gary Kemp and Donald Fagen, for writing such great stories in song. And of course, Tony Hadley.

Thank you to Jesse Larson, the illustrator of my dreams, to April Bamburg, for her editing prowess, and to Bobbi Benson, for making the dream of publication a reality.

Thank you also to my aunt Barbara, who's been my friend as long as she's been my family. And to my children, Griffin and Valerie, along with all my clients, past, present and future — I love you.

Finally, I want to give thanks in triplicate — thank you, thank you, thank you — to my God of Unconditional Love.

She had one idea, and it was... right?

ABOUT THE CREATORS

EMILY SUSSMAN is a licensed clinical social worker and psychotherapist who believes that lavishing your life with love is the best relapse prevention there is. Her outpatient treatment practice, Freedom Recovery Group of South Bend, offers group and individual therapy for adults. She lives in Indiana with her kids, pets, and plants.

J.E. LARSON is the illustrator for the *Secrets of the Ancient Gods* series by Astra Publishing House, and he also illustrates covers for Ransom Note Press. He lives in Minneapolis, Minnesota.

Printed in the USA
CPSIA information can be obtained
at www.ICGtesting.com
LVHW010722110823
754884LV00041B/951

9 798988 478607